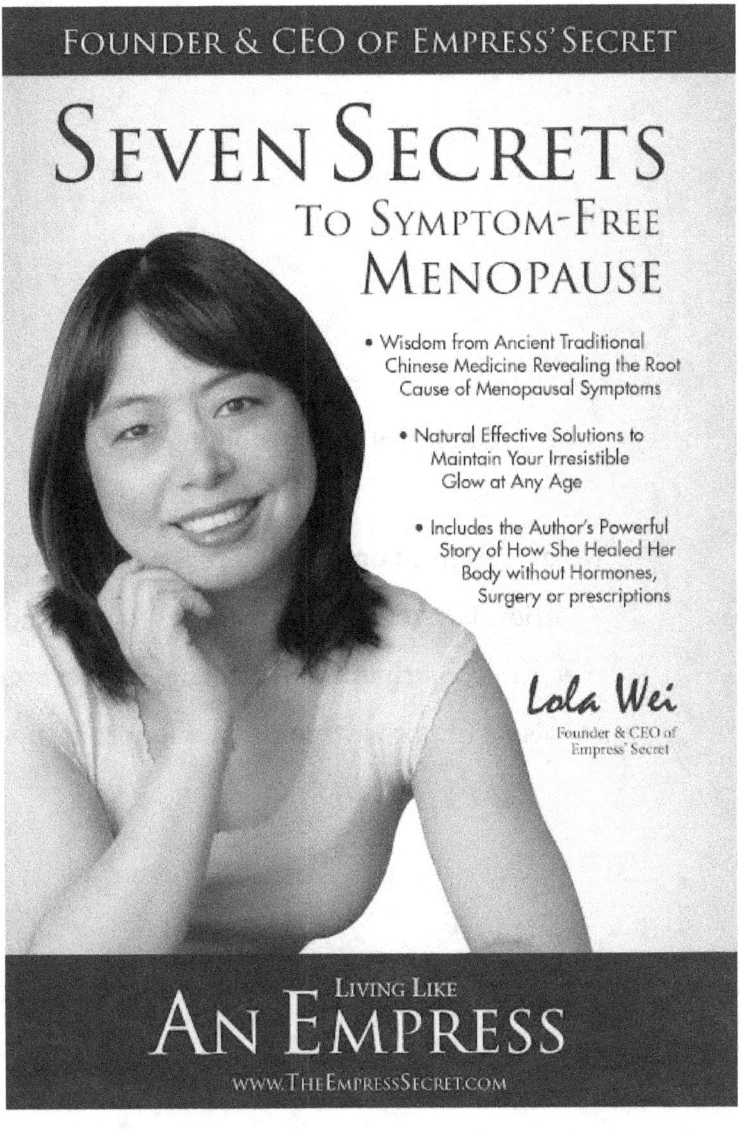

FOUNDER & CEO OF EMPRESS' SECRET

SEVEN SECRETS
TO SYMPTOM-FREE
MENOPAUSE

- Wisdom from Ancient Traditional Chinese Medicine Revealing the Root Cause of Menopausal Symptoms

- Natural Effective Solutions to Maintain Your Irresistible Glow at Any Age

- Includes the Author's Powerful Story of How She Healed Her Body without Hormones, Surgery or prescriptions

Lola Wei

Founder & CEO of
Empress' Secret

LIVING LIKE
AN EMPRESS
WWW.THEEMPRESSSECRET.COM

By Lola Wei

Contents

Why I Wrote This Book

Hello! My name is Lola Wei and I am the Founder of Empress' Secret. I am 45 years young and I feel even healthier and more vibrant than when I was in my 20s and 30s; but it wasn't always that way...

You see, 8 years ago I was in a near-death battle for my life with hyperthyroidism (an incurable autoimmune disease) as well as having a 10-centimeter fibroid in my uterus and an ovarian mass. I was in the early phase of peri-menopause; and was also suffering from terrible insomnia.

As a result of this diagnosis, I had to deal with endless blood tests, ultra sound tests, MRIs, X-rays and more. There were moments I thought I was going to die.

I was a single mom of a 2 year old son living here in the United States and all of my family was in China. I felt lonely, scared, abandoned, and hopeless.

I was constantly worried whether I should entrust someone to take care of my son, or if I should send him back to China so I could die alone. The thought that he might grow up without me was unbearable and painful.

Today, 8 years later, I am completely healed from my hyperthyroidism, and my thyroid is intact.
I am fibroid-free, and my uterus and ovaries are also intact.

I sleep like a baby every night and I wake up naturally every morning without ever needing an alarm, feeling vibrant, rested and blessed.

I haven't taken any medication or supplements for over seven years.

I don't have menstrual cramps like I had in my 20s and 30s. In those days I could barely even get out of bed during the first couple of days of my period, since cramps were hitting me like they were going to kill me. Today, at 45, my period is as smooth as a pleasant evening breeze; in fact I hardly notice that it's here. I don't have PMS mood swings at all. My hormones are abundant and balanced, and my body sings like a symphony.

I am doing things that I was not able to do in my 20s, such as ice-skating for three hours immediately after four hours hiking at an elevation of 800 feet.

My skin is as smooth and as soft as a baby's.

The only health issue I had in the past seven years was that three years ago, at my annual check-up, I had an abnormal pap-smear. I chose not to go with what the doctor recommended -- minor surgery to cut off the cervical tissues. I simply continued strengthening my body's immune system. At the six-month follow up, my pap-smear had returned to normal all by itself! My body had healed the abnormal tissue naturally.

So you may be wondering what I did, exactly what took care of all my health issues.

You are about to learn the most powerful and the most incredible secrets about your body. With that knowledge, you will be able to heal almost anything that you may be experiencing or suffering!

Hold your breath, and let's start the journey.

Why You Should Read This Book

If you are in menopause or are approaching menopause (or someone close to you is) and you want to take control of your own health naturally, without hormones, prescription pills, or invasive surgeries and are determined not to let menopause jeopardize the quality of your life for years to come... then this book is for you.

I wrote this book for women who want to say No to menopause and reclaim their power and their health back!

Disclosure

This book is not intended for any diagnostic or medical purpose. It should not be used to replace any medical advice from your doctors.

Everything I am saying here is my personal experience, understanding from my vast research, and my insights from diving into more than 300 ancient TCM books that were all written from thousands to hundreds of years ago.

I am not a medical practitioner. Everything I am sharing with you here is:

Wisdom about TCM's (Traditional Chinese Medicine) holistic perspective about the body and healing is based on Nei Jing and other top TCM authorships.

How TCM's principles have been confirmed and proven to be true based on my personal healing journey from my incurable disease and multiple other health issues to today's radiant health.

My up-close and personal experiences with all my female friends about their struggles with their own female health issues.

Wisdoms from Nei Jing, the most authoritative Traditional Chinese Medicine book written in the ancient language.
The authority of Nei Jing can be summarized as follows:

- The most prominent TCM doctors in China once said that if you don't read the Nei Jing, you should not practice TCM.
- It is the foundation of all TCM, explaining exactly how our body resonates with the universe. Essentially all the organs in the body have to work in harmony so your body can sing like a symphony.

My Healing Journey from an Incurable Disease

When I was first diagnosed with hyperthyroidism, I didn't really think it was a big deal. (Note: Hyperthyroidism, often referred to as overactive thyroid, is a condition that the thyroid gland produces too much of the hormone thyroxin, which can accelerate the body's metabolism significantly and could cause danger if left untreated.)

I had lost nearly 20 pounds in just a few weeks, and my heart palpitations were serious. The doctor gave me the prescription drug Tapozole, which relieved my symptoms.

My endocrinologist told me that there was a good chance that with this medication I could get remission from the condition. I was quite encouraged by that message at the beginning. I never imagined that I would be obliged to take the medication for the rest of my life. , since I was still only in my late 30s. There was no reason for me to believe anything else.

But after a year of taking the medication, I did not see any hope of stopping it. When I asked my endocrinologist how many patients are ever able to stop taking the medication, the answer was, very few. I almost felt betrayed, because he had never told me this. I regretted blindly taking his words in such a naïve way.

The fact is that almost all hyperthyroidism patients end up having their thyroids killed permanently by using radioactive iodine. (Radioactive iodine, typically given in a capsule, is absorbed and concentrated specifically by the thyroid gland.) This treatment destroys thyroid tissue completely. Then the patients have to take artificial thyroid hormones for the rest of their lives.

Hyperthyroidism Affects More Women Than Men

When I mentioned to my female colleagues that I had hyperthyroidism, I was shocked to discover that majority of my female colleagues had the same problem. They all reassured me that it wasn't all that serious to kill the thyroid; they told me they felt normal after radiation, and that taking the artificial thyroid hormone presented little inconvenience, just a pill a day.

The fact that many women share this problem prompted me to do some research and find some statistics about the condition. It startled me that hyperthyroidism is very common in women, especially for those over 30 after giving birth, and it often accompanies other gynecological problems as well.

I began to realize that the chance of getting off the medication was almost zero, given my findings from the research. At that point I knew that my health problem was serious, much more serious than I had thought.

I knew in my heart that I did not want to kill my thyroid.

I knew in my heart that I did not want to take a pill for the rest of my life

No, never! I did not want to do that.

Desperate to Heal

Little did I know that the hyperthyroidism was just the beginning of the downward spiral of my health.

In the same year, I was also found to have a uterine fibroid; it was about 3 cm in diameter, not considered very serious at that point. An ovarian mass was also detected during an ultra-sound exam, so my gynecologist strongly recommended for me to have surgery to remove my ovaries. I was very reluctant to undergo surgery. At one point my doctor even warned me that I was heading on the road to death because of the potential danger of ovarian cancer. My periods were spotty and scattered. I didn't even feel like a woman.

I was desperate to try anything that could convey even just a tiny ray of hope.

I was so desperate that one time I ordered some herbal extract from Canada for more than $500, which turned out to be two bottles of the most disgusting tasting thing I had ever tasted. And of course it did not work.

The biggest lesson that I learned during those desperate times was, when you don't have good health, nothing means anything to you anymore, not your money, not your career, not your work, or any of your physical possessions. I was willing to trade everything I had, every penny I had, to get my good health back.

In the meantime, I invested a lot of time and effort researching every source I could find: the Internet, library, workshops, and bookstores, etc. and trying to find out answers for my deteriorating health.

I began to recognize certain things such as diet, lifestyle and tremendous stress as directly contributing to the rapid decline of my health prior to my diagnosis:

- I had never been a big coffee drinker, but about a year before I was diagnosed with hyperthyroidism, I was working at an office that served coffee daily, and I found it convenient to grab a cup at work every morning. I also frequently had fast food for breakfast and lunch.

- I fell in love with bacon, and I ate it a lot in the months leading up to my diagnosis with hyperthyroidism. I found myself often having ham and other processed meats almost daily.

- I had stopped working out routinely, as I used to do. I told myself that it was because being a single mom was all-consuming, and my new job was very demanding. I didn't realize that I had become complacent. It never occurred to me that not working out on a regular basis could have any impact on me.

I was also under unusually severe stress: I was laid off twice within 12 months; I had to relocate to a new city where I didn't know a soul. I lost the support group and network that I had previously enjoyed. Adjusting to the new city, parting with old friends, leaving my son with my mom in China, and stuck in a house declining in value day by day due to the housing crisis, etc. all of these had their effects on me.

My diet, lifestyle, the tremendous stress from work and emotional distress took a major toll on my health at that time.

I made drastic change on my diet and lifestyle with determination and discipline. The diet and lifestyle changes, combined with the prescription medication, definitely helped stabilize my symptoms. My hyperthyroidism was under control. But my uterine fibroid was growing at an alarming speed: within a year, it grew from 3 cm to almost 8 cm. When I put my hands on my lower abdomen, I could feel a big solid thing inside my belly that was the size of a goose egg.

I was bleeding very heavily during my period every month. In fact, I had to ask a friend to check on me constantly, because I was concerned that I might hemorrhage to death.

I was getting to a point that I had to do something drastic.

My endocrinologist suggested that I go through radiation to kill my thyroid, as medication was not sustainable. He had to order blood work every three months to ensure that my liver was not being damaged by the medication. He told me very explicitly that if my blood work showed signs of damage, I would need to go through the radiation immediately. It was very scary.

My gynecologist suggested that I have a hysterectomy to remove my ovaries and uterus to take care of the fibroid. Since I already had a child, she figured I probably would not want to have any more.

I was barely 40 years old. I just could not accept the fact that I was going to cut out so many organs from my body at such young age. What did I have left? What else would I have to cut out later?

I always believed that everything in our body has its purpose and use. This is my body, my temple. God has a purpose for every single organ there.

I was sure that I did not want to lose any of my organs, but I had no better alternatives. I felt hopeless, frustrated, depressed, and disappointed.

None of the doctors could explain to me why and how I got my disease in the first place. I am sure a lot of people had the same levels of stress that I was experiencing, but not every 38-year-old woman suffered from as many problems as I did.

My gynecologist said, "We know your fibroids are there, but we don't know why."

My endocrinologist said, "It is quite common at your age for women to have hyperthyroidism, we don't know why, but we can take care of it by killing the thyroid."

I began to wonder, if no one could tell me why I had so many problems in the first place, what if I had other problems after the surgery? What if a new problem appeared somewhere else? I was sure the new problems would not be where my organs had already been removed, but in other places.

If I didn't know the root cause of how I got so sick in the first place, I was definitely heading to a point where I would not have anything left to be surgically removed. I was in a very frustrating struggle, and a very hopeless situation.

I was crying out for answers. Why has all this happened to me? I knew I did not want surgery, but I did not know what else could take care of the problems.

In one of the many frustrating conversations with my brother in China, he suggested that he send me some ancient Traditional Chinese Medicine books from my great grandpa. Those books were all written hundreds or thousands of years ago, drawing on wisdoms dating back to Ancient Traditional Chinese Medicine. My brother thought maybe I could go through them to see if the ancient wisdom might offer some help.

I Found Answers!

I didn't know that my life was about to change completely.

Growing up in a family with generations of Traditional Chinese herbalists, TCM had always been a familiar yet distant subject; I have many memories of my mother brewing fresh ginger tea to treat stomach cramps, the unique scent of my grandpa's herbal brew, and the grass-like herbs used in cooking. These were all faint memories that were about to become the bedrock of my battle plan.

When I was in elementary and middle school, my teacher of ancient Chinese Literature never told us that if you mastered the ancient language you would have the key to unlock the hidden treasures and wisdom found in the ancient books. Little did I know that my straight "A"s in Ancient Chinese Literature would allow me to dive into all the ancient Chinese herbal wisdom with passion.

I was soaking up the ancient TCM like a sponge!

I was enlightened by the philosophy of Traditional Chinese Medicine, which is based on the belief that everything in the universe is interdependent and mutually interactive. Human beings are part of this holistic entity and should be understood with reference to the whole.

I was deeply rooted in the concept that our body works as a unified system, rather than a collection of independent organs. This concept is the reason why certain inherited weaknesses can contribute to a later predisposition to certain diseases.

I found out that the heavy stress and life-changing events had taken a major toll on my body, and directly contributed to my downward spiral of health.

I also learned that for women, any unresolved and accumulated stress and anger eventually show up in gynecological problems through stagnated liver *Qi*. Any emotional turbulence causes the liver to stagnate significantly as well, which gradually affects our entire body.

Qi, in Traditional Chinese Medicine, Qi (also called Qi, Chi or Ki) often translated as "life force", or "energy flow" or "natural energy", is an active principal forming part of any living thing, the central underlying principle in Traditional Chinese Medicine.

The liver is the most important organ for women. Emotional stress will cause the liver Qi to stagnate. Any accumulated anger, extended period of depression, unresolved emotional trauma, unspeakable pain, or heavy levels of stress, etc. will make the liver more and more sluggish, and ultimately affect the menstrual cycle, libido, sleep quality, reproductive system and the autoimmune system.

The liver has its own ways, within limits, to rejuvenate itself and to break down stress and sluggishness. For example, routine physical exercise will help the liver to break down toxins and eliminate them through perspiration. The elevated levels of adrenaline from being constantly exposed to fight-mode can be broken down from intensive physical workouts as well. It is one of the ways that our body is designed to self-rejuvenate via the liver, and help to relieve accumulated stress. Perspiration from working out, from aerobic exercises, from oxygen-rich outdoor activities, will eliminate a lot of toxins from our body.

When our body's internal Qi is compromised from external factors, such as stress, emotional turbulence, or an unhealthy diet and lifestyle, our immune system is also deeply affected, leaving our body more vulnerable to attack from certain diseases.

For example, if two people were to go through the same stressful situation or life changing events, chances are that they could sooner or later develop totally different diseases resulting from the extended period of stressful situations.

In my case, I had an autoimmune endocrine disease and gynecological problems. Another person could develop rheumatoid arthritis, or chronic sinusitis, or joint problems. It all depends on how we were born, with the uneven strength of all the organs in our individual body related to the five elements of TCM at the first point.

The Five Elements, or Five Phases, are five aspects of Qi. In Traditional Chinese Medicine, the Five Elements are wood, fire, earth, metal and water, the five primary aspects of Qi.

In the poetic language of the Five Elements, health is a harmonious balance of all the elements. The Qi of the five elements ebbs and flows in daily and seasonal cycles. Each one of us is a unique and characteristic blend of the influences of all the elements.

The findings were enlightening, encouraging, and gave me hope.

I finally figured out why I was having so many health issues, one by one, seemingly never-ending. Clearly my body was not born with strong in-born Qi or life force. Over the years, my Qi was depleted much more rapidly because of giving birth, post-maternity heavy stress from work and an unusually chaotic life, natural aging, life-changing events, diet and lifestyle, etc...

There is solution for every disease

The most encouraging thing was that there was a solution...

Nei Jing, also known as *The Yellow Emperor's Inner Classic*, is one of the most important classics of Taoism, and the highest authority on TCM (Traditional Chinese Medicine). It has been documented that Nei Jing was written by the great Huang Di, the Yellow Emperor, who reigned during the third millennium BCE.

According to Nei Jing, the highest authority of TCM, there is so-called in-born Qi, which we all have and carry along throughout our lives; there is also Acquired Qi, which can be replenished and boosted through food, herbs, proper nutrition, etc. that can help you build your body back to its optimal level of self-rejuvenation and self-healing.

Not everyone is created equal in terms of in-born Qi. Some of us have more, some of us have less. Some of us are naturally born strong with good health, while some of us are naturally born a bit weak with average or sub-par health. Yet, there is a way and opportunity for us to replenish and strengthen our body with more acquired Qi so our longevity is extended and our aging curve smoothed out. If we know how to nurture our body with what it needs and let our body work following the law of nature, then our body will heal anything that does not belong naturally and bring itself back to its healthy state.

The most difficult part of this process is how to give our body what it needs effectively and efficiently. Often we hear people say that they eat a healthy diet and work out diligently every day, yet still do not feel as good as they want to, or still get sick. Sometimes they even contract diseases that Western medicine can treat only with surgery.

The human body is such a sophisticated system, that it remains a mystery to even modern science, let alone to most people. There are more and more studies supporting the theory that our body's self-healing power is beyond what we can ever imagine. The power of our mind and attitudes is also beyond what we can ever imagine.

First Success: Healing from Hyperthyroidism

I started making my own elixir based on the most classic yet very simple Traditional Chinese Medicine formulation that has been used and documented for thousands of years to replenish and strengthen my body with this acquired, boosted life force Qi. The formula itself only contains three primary ingredients that have been prescribed by hundreds of top TCM herbalists throughout TCM's history to boost the body's Qi and immune system so the body will have the resources to tackle chronic diseases.

After six weeks of my self-made TCM treatment, I felt great and was getting better and better. So I started gradually reducing my medication, as the first step of healing process is to make my body function normally. I first started with cutting the dosage in half, making sure my symptoms were stable and that my body did not have any drastic reaction to the reduced dosage. Success! Then as I continued drinking the potion to strengthen my body's Qi, I gradually reduced the dosage further, from half to a quarter size of my original dosage, and eventually completely stopped the medication altogether.

It was a long process; it took me about three or four months to completely come off the medication. The moment when I did not have any noticeable symptoms without any medication, I knew the healing was working, and my body was recovering.

On my next follow-up doctor's visit, the blood work of my entire thyroid index had returned to normal, except for my TSH (TSH: Thyroid-Stimulating Hormone, is a major thyroid health function index in blood tests for thyroid function) that was still very high. The doctor announced that I was officially in remission, though he never asked me what I did. He probably thought it just got to remission all by itself. He told me the TSH typically takes much longer to get back to normal but I was definitely on the right track.

It has been eight years now and my thyroid has been functioning perfectly, without any recurrence at all. My doctor told me that the longer I could stay in remission, the less likely the disease would come back.

Healing Uterine Fibroids

With regard to my uterine fibroid, I ultimately decided to undergo myomectomy surgery rather than a full hysterectomy to remove just the fibroid tumor, preserving all my reproductive organs. It was not an easy choice, but I made it through and recovered perfectly.

My ovarian mass turned out to be a massive fibroid tumor that was quite aggressive. To be able to preserve my uterus and ovaries while surgically removing just the tumor was a miracle. It took determination and relentless efforts, and superior skill and expertise of the doctor to make it happen.

Equipped with wisdom about how our body works, I was determined to give my body a second chance to rebuild my health after the surgery. I vowed that I would never again take my health for granted and do everything I could to lead a healthy and vibrant life. Since then I had continued to enjoy transformative health like never before. I feel like I am aging in reverse! I am doing things now in my forties that I could never do in my twenties. My energy is boundless!

I just want to assure you that you can do the same too no matter what health problems you are currently suffering. If you are healthy and young, you will be very blessed to be equipped with this knowledge and wisdom so you will never let any health issues drag down your quality of life.

Empress' Secret - Glow Was Born

So now you know my story. It is because of what I experienced that I founded the Empress' Secret. It is the passion of sharing this treasured wisdom about living a radiant health life in the most sustainable and effortless way that led me on this journey.

Before I created the Glow, I had been using the same nourishing ingredients myself for years and have been benefited tremendously. All the ingredients such as Jujube Dates, Goji Berry, Lotus Seeds and Dragon Eye Fruits are all super foods on earth and they have tremendous nutrients compared to other typical fruits we normally consume. I used to brew the delicious and nutritious tonic from these rare roots and super fruits in my coffee pot, and then pouring the tonic in bottles and carry it with me to gym and to work. This way I could consume the tonic daily to nourish and replenish my body and build up more reserve of my Qi. I also brewed it often for my friends coming over for a visit.

To actually make Empress' Secret - Glow available as a shelf stable tonic drink was a daunting task, especially I wanted to make it as pure as the Mother Nature offers with no sugar no sweetener added, no preservative and no artificial flavoring at all. But it happened so effortlessly with the Lord opening the doors to make the impossible possible.

I feel very humbled and privileged to have the opportunity to do something for others. I always tell people I make Glow, and I drink Glow myself every day. It is nothing but a gift. Even the distributor and the limited retail stores carrying it told me that there is nothing like Glow in the market because it is almost not commercially viable to make something like Glow. As much as I am proud of making Empress' Secret Glow so pure the way as I wanted, I feel humbled for this opportunity that many people will have chance to experience the wisdom and benefits from Traditional Chinese Medicine.

Aging is a natural process, and we cannot stop it, but we can slow it down. We can renew ourselves. We can rejuvenate ourselves. We can make our aging curve much smoother.

Like the mythical phoenix bird, our bodies have the natural ability to renew themselves. This drink was created to be the key to unlock your body's rejuvenating system, so that you too can experience radiant health.

Today, I feel very blessed and very fortunate. If I had followed what the doctors said, I would have lost my thyroid, uterus, ovaries, and who knows what else.

I am glad I did not give up seeking out a solution of healing myself. Every single event that happened in my life played a crucial role in transforming me into what I am today. My gratitude is beyond what words can describe. I have learned never to take my health for granted. I continue to nurture my body carefully and expect to enjoy today's radiant health for many years to come.

I hope you feel inspired to take charge of your own health, and I wish you vibrant health and effortless longevity. I am sure you will with the treasured wisdom revealed to you here. You will be empowered to achieve sustained beauty and vitality in the most effortless way while aging gracefully.

About Nei Jing

As I mentioned earlier, Nei Jing, also known as *The Yellow Emperor's Inner Classic*, is one of the most important classics of Taoism, and the highest authority on traditional Chinese medicine. It has been documented that Nei Jing was written by the great Huang Di, the Yellow Emperor, who reigned during the third millennium BCE.

Nei Jing contains a total of eighty-one chapters known as the *Suwen,* or "Questions of Organic and Fundamental Nature.", a foundation of Chinese life sciences and medicine.

Nei Jing's fundamental concept is based on how natural law works. It uses the *yin/yang* and Five Elements doctrines to define health and disease, and repeatedly emphasizes personal responsibility for the length and quality of one's life.

Nei Jing encompasses etiology, physiology, diagnosis, therapy, and prevention of disease, as well as in-depth investigation of such diverse subjects as ethics, psychology, and cosmology. All of these subjects are discussed in a holistic context that says life is not fragmented, as in the model provided by modern science, but rather that all the pieces make up an interconnected whole. By revealing the natural laws of this holistic universe, the book offers the most comprehensive, in-depth and practical advice on how to promote a long, happy, and healthy life.

It is thought that Nei Jing was compiled roughly two thousand years ago, building on the Yellow Emperor's original work; it is believed that all TCM's significant medical works were based on or tremendously benefited from the enlightenment of this unparalleled book.

Although TCM philosophy has over 5000 years of history since the origin of China, the earliest systematic compilation of its theory and fundamental views and treatments were documented roughly 2000-4000 years ago.

World-famous medical masters and saints in the history of TCM, such as Zhang Zhongjing, Hua Tuo, Sun Simiao and Li Shizhen, who lived hundreds of years ago, were greatly enlightened by The Medical Classic of the Yellow Emperor. All of them mastered the essence of this book, thus becoming the most famous practitioners of TCM in Chinese history.

This book not only saved my life, but also changed my life forever

There are no words that can describe the deep gratitude I have for my capability of reading through and fully understanding the context of this great work. I feel blessed that I was able to apply my knowledge to my own body and to heal myself.

Today, I am privileged to have the opportunity to share what I have learned with you, so you don't have to go through what I did, and you can live a life with sustained beauty, vitality and longevity in the most effortless way.

If you have chance to read this book, hold your breath; I am just about to reveal some of the most treasured, yet hidden wisdom about your body and your health.

Before we start with the seven secrets, there are some very important TCM fundamentals that you need to know so that you will have a much deeper understanding of all the secrets I am revealing.

TCM Fundamentals and its Holistic View

TCM is a complete healing philosophy whose principles and theories have existed for thousands of years.

TCM believes that everything in the universe is interdependent and mutually interactive. Our body is a small universe, just like the macro universe, and should be analyzed with reference to the whole. For example, if you have menopausal symptoms, most likely that problem is attributed to your internal Qi deficiency and liver sluggishness from accumulated emotional distress.

If your period continues longer than five to seven days and you experience spotting between periods, chances are that your Liver Qi and Spleen Qi are both deeply weakened, and are thus unable to regulate the normal ending of the bleeding.

If you have skin problems, be it rash or acne, most likely it is related to lung Qi deficiencies.

Essentially, all the organs have to work in harmony in order to absorb the nutrients from what you eat and drink. The spleen Qi energy is the fundamental life force and manifests the entire digestive system.

Spleen Qi is Fundamental for Your Health

We all know there are millions of health products, such as raw, fermented juice, smoothies, veggie extracts, etc.; however, if you are deficient in spleen Qi energy, not only will you be unable to absorb the nutrients, but the raw harsh food could further compromise your body. Because your body has to work much harder to digest raw foods, it depletes more Qi, the life force, from your spleen. As a consequence, your body will not completely take in the nutrients from raw foods; additionally it could weaken your Spleen Qi even further.

Think about it: we are not living in tribal times anymore with our primary diet on raw foods. We are living in modern society. We are so used to eating mostly cooked foods, so our digestive system is already very well adapted to the modern diet.

Some people think we should go back to all raw veggies. It is absolutely true, there are more nutrients and live enzymes in raw foods, but is your body equipped to handle them? For sure, your body can digest much more if you are in your 20s, when it works at its prime level with strong internal Qi and all organs rejuvenating at an optimal level.

When you were in your 20s, even if you partied hard all night long, only slept two or three hours, you woke up fine, no dark circles under your eyes and not feeling tired at all; you were just like the morning sun, vibrant and shining effortlessly with no need for any external help.

Then, what happens after you turn 30, or even 40? You can't sleep well; you can't party all night, because aging will show immediately on your face, and you don't have much energy the next day.

As we age, our internal Qi naturally declines; this is the natural course that no one can stop. But, we can either preserve our internal Qi through a healthy lifestyle, or we can replenish our body with more Acquired Qi to sustain the aging curve much more smoothly. That is how and why TCM works, because it has time-tested recipes from super foods and rare roots to give your body the fundamental boost to replenish and strengthen your Qi, provide you with more Acquired Qi so you can reverse aging and increase longevity and vitality.

This explains why for some people, even if they do everything right, eat a healthy diet and work out diligently, they still don't feel as good as they want to or used to be because their bodies are not taking in the nutrients from what they eat and drink as effectively and efficiently as before. Without boosting their fundamental Spleen Qi to bring their digestive function to its optimal level, whatever they are doing will be compromised.

Once you start to apply this principle and focus on boosting your fundamental Spleen Qi, so that you can absorb nutrients more efficiently, your whole body in turn will work like a symphony! A lot of miraculous things will happen in an effortless way because your body will be healing, rejuvenating and restoring itself.

Let Your Body Heal Itself

Another TCM principle is to let food be your medicine. TCM doctors consider the top healing herbs as edible food with tremendous natural healing properties that provide everyday nutrients to nurture the body.

The law of nature is to let your body work. When you nourish your body with what it needs, it will eliminate all toxins and heal itself. The food you take in either nurtures you or depletes you.

TCM believes that everyone is born with the ability to self-heal, especially women. The uterus and ovaries have a unique capability of healing themselves, and helping the body to restore healthy functions.

TCM believes that healthy women have the capacity to generate enough hormones for their entire life. Even if the hormones may not as high as they were during a woman's child-bearing years, it will be enough to last her for the rest of her life.

TCM does not diagnose any isolated medical complaints. For example, if women have excessive menstrual bleeding, or spotting between periods, or an extended period with non-stop bleeding, it is not actually a physical uterine or lining problem, the problem is most likely connected to sluggishness of the liver and spleen Qi deficiency, as they are so weakened that they cannot regulate the bleeding.

TCM is beyond scientific and measurable. Its foundation is deeply rooted in understanding Qi and our body as an inseparable energy system. Each individual part of this energy system is communicating and interacting with all the other parts in a constant state.

TCM sees and treats the whole person from all aspects encompassing body, mind, emotion, and spirit for lasting health and longevity.

The self-healing technique of TCM can make a major impact on women's health in western society.

Here are seven absolutely incredible and best-treasured secrets you need to know about menopause, so you can have a trouble-free menopausal transitional time for the years to come. Even if you are currently suffering from menopausal symptoms, you can use the bonus tips at the end of this book to start transforming your life forever. I have friends who used the formula to completely eliminate hormone replacement therapy in just 7 days. The miracle formula will help relieve your symptoms like a wonder fountain of youth. I just want you to be assured that your life will never be the same.

Introduction of Women's Life Cycles

Before we go into these secrets, let's talk about how women's body age based on the TCM view.

According to Nei Jing, women have seven-year cycles—like the phases of the progressed moons such as the new moon, half-moon and full moon.

Women's cycles start with the first seven years, during which a healthy young girl's kidney Qi will manifest the growth of her hair and permanent teeth. At the second seven year cycle, about 14 years of age, the Qi and life force reaches its peak, causing the arrival of puberty and the beginning of menstrual periods.

A woman blossoms through her fertile years, then at about age 35, the fifth of seven years, her Qi starts to decline, which is part of the natural aging process. No one can stop this process, but how steeply and how rapidly the aging curve declines is totally up to you.

Menopause typically occurs between the sixth and seventh cycles from 42 years old to 49 years old.

TCM believes women's menstrual cycles ending as a natural part of a woman's life, just like there is a beginning and an end for any cycle.

The #1 Secret: Menopausal Symptoms Are Not the Result Of Aging, But The Condition Of Your Body Long Before Menopause Begins.

If you are a woman, I would strongly encourage you to print this sentence and hang it somewhere on your board in your office or bedroom to remind yourself that menopausal symptoms are not acceptable conditions for you or for your body. Don't accept menopausal symptoms as normal, just because everyone you know is suffering from them. Don't accept menopausal symptoms as normal, just because the majority of females at that age are experiencing them. .

I hope you have the courage and braveness to say No to symptoms of menopause. Your life is about to change forever from this point on.

<u>Menopause Symptoms</u>

In ancient medical texts, menopause does not appear as a medical word in TCM's dictionary. Menopause is more a western concept and word. TCM recognizes that the menstrual cycle has a beginning and an end, which is nature's way.

During this transitional time, a woman may experience a variety of different problems, if she is not healthy or had not been healthy before reaching this phase.

In other words, if a woman has not been healthy during her 30s, 40s or before menopause, for sure she is going to experience far worse problems as she heads into menopause.

How do we define healthy in this context?

According to TCM views, if a woman's menstrual cycle has always been regular and mostly problem-free, she should not experience a difficult menopause at all.

In an ideal world, if a woman is healthy, her menstruation will be regular and free of any problems. No period cramps, no blood clots, no spotting, no headaches, no migraines, no early or delayed periods, no mood swings. She has always been happy and healthy and her menstrual period has always been smooth, and she does not experience stress from work or family. She is like a beautiful flower blossoming throughout her fertile years, and she will not experience any menopause problems at all.

But in the real world, this is rare. Usually after 35, we feel a lot of things starting their downward spiral. This happens at different speeds for different people. Some of us notice obvious problems, some of us feel a lot of tiny things accumulating in a relatively unnoticeable way, and suddenly, overnight, and we don't feel the same anymore. We are constantly under tremendous pressure -- work, family, children, emotions, spirituality -- and modern society imposes an extremely demanding lifestyle on us. Sometimes we think we are taking good care of ourselves, but we aren't, not because we don't want to, but because we don't know how to. We try to live a healthy lifestyle, we eat right, we work out, yet we are still on this downward spiral. We want to take charge of our own health, yet we don't know how.

We trust our doctors, but they cannot tell us why we got the problems in the first place, and they cannot tell us how to prevent the same problems from coming back.

Most of the time, doctors only help relieve the symptoms, not the actual root cause of our problems.

We constantly face the dilemma of whether to do what doctors say, even when we are not fully convinced that it is in our interest. It is hard; I know. I have been there, I hear you. I thought I was going to die. I never knew I would make it through, much less be where I am today enjoying radiant health. Just imagine, with all the problems we have along the way, we fix one thing, and before we know it, here comes another one.

It seemed nothing really big at the time because I was still young, far away from menopause. We thought we were fine, just a few female problems, and if they are too bothersome, doctors have advanced technologies and surgery to be able to handle them. They can burn the uterus lining to fix heavy bleeding. They can perform a hysterectomy to remove the uterus to take care of endometriosis and uterine fibroids.

Severe Stress Relates to Premature Menopause

When you reach menopause, the entire energy of your body starts a tremendous shift. Bang! Everything suddenly gets a lot worse. Of course, the changes don't happen overnight; they are the result of accumulated effects over an extended time. Now we are trained to believe that serious issues related to menopause are entirely normal!

Say NO! Be brave enough to say No to a difficult menopause!

Now you know, menopause is not really the problem, but the condition of your body before the transition even gets underway.

In my personal experience, almost all my western girlfriends accept difficult menopause as normal because their sisters, their mothers, their friends, their colleagues all experience it. Even doctors tell you that you are getting to that age and are destined to have those problems. The doctors have a solution for you: your female hormones are declining, so you can take Hormone Replacement Therapy (HRT), be it progesterone cream, or an estrogen patch or pill. Even though you feel better, you soon find out you can't live without hormone therapy. If you don't want the HRT, the only other alternative is to deal with the problems on your own.

I started asking my girlfriends if they had any menstrual problems, or other gynecological issues, or severe stress before menopause. It startled me that 100% of the women had menstrual problems, and almost every single woman who had premature menopause before they were 45 years old experienced major life-changing events or were under severe stress, such as divorce, job loss, relocation, family tragedy etc.

Severe stress almost always accompanies premature menopause. This just further confirms and proves that the TCM view that I learned from Nei Jing is so true.

If a woman is in poor health and her internal energy, or Qi, is not balanced or is deficient, her body expresses its condition through many types of menstrual symptoms: premenstrual syndrome (PMS), irregular periods, painful periods, breast tenderness, headaches, cramping, and fever during cramps, to name just a few.

If a woman doesn't suffer from menstrual irregularities during a lifetime of cycles, it is highly unlikely that she will experience difficulties during menopause transitional time; on the other hand, women who have menstrual difficulties on a regular basis are likely to have a difficult menopause.

The reason is simple: their bodies are out of balance and their energy has declined long before they reach menopause.

According to Neil Jing, menopause is one of the biggest transitions of any woman's life. During this period, there is an enormous energy shift within a women's body that goes far beyond physical changes, which is natural and normal.

If you are able to understand this special opportunity and take the time to readjust, replenish, rejuvenate and strengthen your internal Qi, you can help prevent new problems arising from this transitional time. Otherwise, after this turning point, without a sufficient level or reserves of internal Qi, you will not have the strength to deal with many health problems that often come with aging.

As we age, our Qi naturally declines. This means we have less energy to "spend" doing our normal daily routine. If no adjustment is made for this energy "gap," the body and its organs will be affected.

So if you are currently experiencing any menopausal symptoms -- night sweats, thinning hair, hot flashes, lower libido, et --take a deep breath, look back over the past three to seven years of your life to see if you had ignored all the small peri-menopause signs that your body was trying to send you.

You probably tried to take good care of your body, but lack of holistic knowledge and wisdom that truly works may have hindered your efforts to go through a problem-free menopause

It is never too late to take complete charge of your body. With the knowledge you are obtaining from this book, you can rebuild your temple in the most effortless way. I've included a few simple TCM classic herb formulas specifically for women suffering from severe menopausal symptoms. You can make simple home remedies to replenish your body, and you can be assured that you will significantly benefit from these remedies for the rest of your life.

Research and Study on the Epidemic of Difficult Menopause in the Western World

According to an article published in the Huffington Post, researchers from the Department of Integrated Health at Westminster University polled 1,000 British women aged 45 to 55, and compared their answers to those of women from the U.S., Canada, Japan and China. The conclusion was that Japanese and Chinese women suffer the fewest menopausal symptoms. British and American women suffer the most.

Another study published by Pacific College of Oriental Medicine stated the interesting fact that 75% of American women experience noticeable menopausal discomfort, while only 10% of Asian women do. .

For Chinese women, hot flashes and night sweats are very uncommon experiences, and very few use hormone replacement therapy at all.

The truth is that the majority of Asian women never experience the enormous amount of discomfort that American women seem to universally suffer during the menopausal years.

I never remembered my mother experiencing any menopausal problems except for a few minor mood swings and irritability, according to my father. What I do know is my mom never even heard of HRT and very few of her peers ever used HRT at all.

It's worth considering that it is the combination of diet, culture, and Chinese herbs that is the determining factor in maintaining the health of Asian women through menopause.

It is the "Yin" and "Yang", and ultimately, the balance of "Yin" and "Yang", supported by natural foods and herbs rather than HRT that keep your body functioning at the optimal level and achieve sustained health, beauty and happiness.

Traditionally, Asian cultures have long understood that herbs can be added to the daily diet to provide everyday nourishment. For example, Chinese jujube dates are almost every Asian woman's nourishing food, though they are scarcely known in America. Asian women have seen their mothers and grandmothers brewing the jujube dates along with Gobi berry and lotus seeds for their menstrual cramps, or when they give birth. These are the times when their bodies need nutrients the most. The fact is that Asian women are more in tune to their menstrual regularities long before they reach menopause.

Let me give you some examples: I have a few Chinese girlfriends here in the U.S. Whenever they noticed even just a tiny bit of irregularity with their periods, such as blood clots, stomach cramps, migraine, or darkened color, they would go to a Chinese store and get some jujube dates or angelica and start brewing soup every day until their periods had returned to normal.

It is interesting to note that it is very common for Chinese girls to pay a high level of attention to the quality of their period - from the color, mood, body reaction, smoothness, to the length of the period, etc. If they feel they have lost too much blood, they would cook a very nutritious soup to replenish their bodies. Chinese girls would intuitively add some simple roots and herbs to their daily diet to defy aging and to maintain optimal health, as they understand that the principles of nutrition work effectively.

Asian women rarely turn to artificial hormone remedies as American women do. They nourish their bodies with natural plant-based foods, including time -tested TCM herbs.

The #2 Secret: For Women, The Liver Is The Most Important Organ To Help You Achieve Effortless Radiant Health And Longevity.

For women, the liver is the most important organ in regulating your hormones. Your emotional state is directly related to the healthy flow of your Liver Qi, thus the proper functioning of your liver. Liver Qi's Free Flow is crucial in regulating female hormones and the balance of all other organs to keep the harmony of how our bodies function as a whole.

It is often said that stress is a silent killer. This is true. I have first-hand experience to prove that extended exposure to a stressful situation was a primary cause of my multiple gynecological issues.

When I was struggling to heal myself from the series of illnesses, I later recognized that several life-changing events had taken place prior to my initial diagnosis. I had an affair with a married man before I came to America. The hopeless relationship lasted for years until I was fed up and escaped to America, an alien planet to me at the time, given my limited English. I went to business school that meant a very fast-paced and demanding lifestyle. I was dating a rock star for a very short period of time and had a very hard time to adjust to America's social life. I rekindled the affair with my old lover and unexpectedly got pregnant as a single woman. I struggled to give birth to my child and suffered from postpartum depression and dealing with an extremely stressful work situation after my maternity leave. I took a new job and relocated to Reno. I left my then 4-month old son in China with my mother so I could finish moving, selling my house, and buying another house in the new city. Then I was laid off from the new job scarcely four months after I had relocated. I was lucky to get a new job in just two weeks but then I was laid off again 10 months later. I was unemployed for first time in my life. I was a single mother with an infant child, all by myself with my family far away in China. I missed my old friends, I was thinking about moving back, but the housing bubble burst, and I could not sell my house. I was plagued with uncertainties about my future, my life, my son. I lacked my usual supporting network and friends in the new place. I felt stuck in a strange city, I felt abandoned, depressed, disappointed, angry...

Clearly all these stressful events directly contributed to the deterioration of my health, especially since at the time I had reached the age of natural decline, the late 30s.

I had never really taken good care of myself during my 20s and even early 30s; though I thought I was doing just fine, until I was not fine.

My life had always been hectic, fast- paced, yet it never occurred to me that anything was wrong. Looking back, there were a lot of warning signs from the quality of my menstrual cycle, but I never dreamed they would have anything to do with the overall condition of my health.

We are trained to believe that problems with the menstrual cycle are normal; most women have similar problems, so why worry? Then *bang,* all the compounding effects from everything that has been building up strike and you have nowhere to escape. I found myself in a life- or- death situation

It is often said that emotion is women's best friend and worst enemy.
Emotion makes us a woman, yet overwhelming emotion often plays against our very best interests as women. We often let our emotions run over us, preventing us from pursuing our own best interests.

Be aware of the stress and the pressure that you are undergoing from your work, your partner, your marriage, your relationship, and your children, for weeks, months, or even years. There is a reason for everything, yet the most important thing is to learn and to grow from our bad experiences.

According to Nei Jing, the liver rules your psycho-spiritual nature and your emotional state, such as your stress level, your anger, suppressed anger, depression, or any emotional turbulence. All these will directly affect the Liver Qi flow.

It should be noted that the Liver Qi we are talking about here is a completely different concept from the liver function in standard Western Medicine. Western Medicine has no concept of liver Qi Stagnation. Western medicine primarily depends on blood tests of Liver Panel (AST & ALT are the main indexes) to check for any abnormality or major liver damage – such as hepatitis or sclerosis. Chances are that you could have perfectly fine liver panel blood work with very bad liver stagnation symptoms. Your doctor likely will tell you that your liver is fine.

I have never had any abnormal liver panel blood results, yet I had severe liver stagnation symptoms, reflected in my severe gynecological and endocrine problems.

The liver is also responsible for storing and moving the blood and Qi smoothly throughout the body. When Liver Qi is not flowing freely, it becomes sluggish.

Stress, emotional distress and suppressed anger over extended periods of time, as well as the toxicity of modern life (poor diet, chemicals in our food and environment, overwork, etc.) all cause the Liver Qi to stagnate and thus take a toll on the liver. Since the liver plays the central role in the smooth flow of Qi in the body, disharmony of the liver can affect all the other organs. And it could also directly affect your hormone and immune system.

For women, most gynecological related medical problems are directly associated with Liver Qi stagnation, because the liver is directly responsible for the regularity, volume and flow of the menstrual cycle. Anything that disrupts the smooth flow of liver energy is likely to have a negative impact on menstruation, reproductive health, and libido and later aggravate menopause symptoms.

In addition to obvious menstrual disorders, Liver Qi stagnation can also cause spasms, migraines, tendinitis, hypertension, irritability or depression, anger disorders, moodiness, pain, endometriosis, reproductive abnormalities, low or none libido, etc.

I have read more than 300 ancient TCM books and they all emphasize how important liver stagnation is to women's health.

In Western society, most people do not automatically connect female problems with the liver. Yet, if you ask all the women who suffer from severe gynecological problems -- including cancer, extreme stress and unexpected life-changing events -- were almost always present before those problems became too big to ignore.

TCM believes that cancer takes between four and forty years to develop. Cancer tumors do not develop overnight except those specific cases triggered by nuclear, chemical or environmental poisons.

It is significant that Western people don't typically realize that certain conditions, such as problematic periods, are warning signs about your body's internal imbalance. Given proper nutritional and stress management support on a timely basis, those problems could very easily be resolved and prevent other more severe problems, such as menopausal difficulties – even breast cancer or uterine cancer -- from appearing in later years.

When your menstrual period is not regular or problem-free, chances are your immune system is also compromised, leaving the door open for other diseases to attack. This is very important.

You need to take control of your own emotional state, because regardless of how perfect an herb formula is, if your emotional state is not being aware, properly managed to have it under control, it is likely that medical complaints will return, as the root cause has not been addressed.

TCM recognizes that lifestyle has a significant influence on whether a woman will have a difficult menopause or not. A woman with a long-standing pattern of anxiety, depression, stress, poor diet, addictions and overwork is more predisposed to a difficult menopause (or difficult menstrual periods) than someone who leads a more balanced and moderate lifestyle.

Unfortunately, we live in a hectic society that doesn't readily lend itself to balance and harmony without a good bit of effort. We eat irregularly, experience stress, do not allow for enough rest and exercise and frequently run on empty stomach. Chronic fatigue is one result and so is a difficult menopause.

The good news is that there are time-tested Chinese herbs and classic TCM formulas that can be very effective at relieving the physical and emotional symptoms of menopause by soothing the liver Qi, strengthening spleen and kidney functions and calming the mind and spirit. However, as mentioned previously, you need to take control of your own emotional state, because regardless of how perfect an herb formula can be, if your emotional state is not under control, it will not be effective.

According to Heritage from Fu Qing Zhu About Women's Issues, most medical issues of women can be addressed through treating irregularities of menstrual cycle, because for women, it is all about blood Qi and Liver Qi balance and harmony. This book also states that, for women who have stopped menstrual cycles, most medical complaints can be addressed through strengthening the Spleen Qi to boost the digestive system, as the Spleen Qi manifests how the entire body functions. Maintaining a strong Spleen Qi is fundamental for extending longevity.

Starting today, I encourage you to listen to your body, to pay more attention and be more in tune to your own body, especially your periods. Pay attention to your body's reaction before, during and after the period. Start developing your own ritual to take care of your body, especially during your period, avoid strenuous physical work, relax and rest more during those times, treat yourself like a queen, pamper yourself, cook nutritious soups to replenish your body, listen to music, take the day off if you can, and just spoil yourself.

It is often said that women are like tidal waves, with its ebb and flow. Our period is like the ebb: the better care and rest you give to your body, the bigger tidal wave is going to come afterwards, with more vibrant energy, balanced moods, and happiness and joyfulness so you can enjoy life to the fullest.

It is not hard once you learn and understand the way to take care of your body properly, and can be very simply done by adding nutrient-rich food to your daily diet.

Other than severe stress and distressed emotional states, common factors causing Liver Qi Stagnation are:

- **Drugs**. The first and foremost is drugs, including all pharmaceutical medications and over-the-counter pills. All pills require the liver to break them down, so they can get into the bloodstream of your body to have the desired effect. When the liver breaks down these drugs, it adds extra stress and leaves more toxins in your body, which will require the liver to work much harder to eliminate. So next time you pick up ibuprofen from over the counter, think again: is the pain a warning signal that your body is trying to show you, or do you want to use the pain killer to mask the warning sign and ignore the root cause?

- **Other common toxins include:**

  - Coffee
  - Alcohol
  - Sugar
  - Soda pop
  - Pollutants: environmental, chemical, etc.
  - Excessive hormones (one of the main jobs of the liver is to clear hormones from the blood)

Certain people could have other sensitivities (that act like toxins to your liver) to such as dairy products or wheat or others.

The #3 Secret: Make a Fully Informed Decision About Any Reproductive Surgery and Preserve Your Ovary Whenever You Can

Just because you no longer desire to have children does not mean your female organs are no longer useful. I would encourage you to keep all your female organs, especially your ovaries, from being surgically removed whenever you can or medically allowed.

I hope you would never accept undergoing an elective hysterectomy.

If you are like me, with uterine fibroids, I would encourage you to be brave enough to tell your doctor that you want to keep all your female organs intact and only remove the tumors.

Medically, it is completely possible with today's non-invasive robot-assisted Da Vinci surgery. Yes, it is more complicated and requires sophisticated skills, but you can make it happen because after all, it is your own body!

When my uterine fibroid grew from 3 cm to almost 10 cm, it became a huge burden in my life, both physically and emotionally. My period was miserable and horrendous at the time with the huge fibroid inside my uterus; I would bleed non-stop for seven to ten days, with huge blood clots. Literally I thought I would die from such heavy periods any month. I was very anemic, and my hemoglobin level was dangerously low.

But I was still very reluctant to have my uterus surgically removed. I just wanted to have myomectomy (removing only the fibroid). I did not want to have a hysterectomy, which is what my gynecologist recommended…

I literally visited more than 20 gynecologists in my small town; there did not seem be any options other than the hysterectomy.

I was so frustrated that at one of the gynecologist's office, I broke down and cried. I still remember his name was Bethel, the House of God. I loved him dearly. He was warm- hearted, nice, and compassionate. He saw me in his office, not in a regular examination room.

He looked into my eyes saying, "You know that you will die if you don't do anything, regardless of how much you don't want to. You have to do something with your tumor, do you understand?" I was crying like a baby. He gave me a hug and said, "If you really want to keep your uterus, what we can do is just get the fibroid out, but it is major surgery, like a C-section, and since your blood level is so low, there is the risk that you might die from excessive blood loss during the surgery." I felt scared and helpless.

Nevertheless, I was prepared to have major surgery to just remove the fibroid while keeping my uterus intact. But I was still relentlessly searching for any other possible non-invasive option for having myomectomy. Then the miracle happened...

Again, my extensive research efforts paid off. At that time, Robot-Assisted Da Vinci surgery for gynecology was still quite new, though it had been used for a while for cardiovascular surgery and other medical fields. There were only three gynecologists trained to perform the Da Vinci non-invasive surgery, and to perform it on myomectomy surgery, it was still very new and it requires at least two trained surgeons to be present. Only one of them had done similar myomectomy. Others had done hysterectomy. I visited all three of them and consulted them with my long list of questions about the surgery.

Finally, after watching the entire surgery performed by Michigan University Hospital on internet, I decided to do the non-invasive Robot-Assisted Da Vinci surgery to remove my fibroid while keeping my uterus intact.

The surgery went very successfully, and I recovered very well too though I had to have blood transfusion before the surgery due to my severe anemia. I know in my heart that it was God's mercy and grace leading me to accomplish all this. It was a second chance I was given to rebuild my life. My gratitude was beyond that words can describe.

A sharp contrast from my case is: one of my close friends Sandra, who was in her early 50s, had a huge ovarian cyst that caused tremendous pain. Since her doctor was afraid it was ovarian cancer, she was referred to an oncologist, who told her that the solution was to have a hysterectomy so to eliminate any risk of cancer. Luckily, the pathology test showed the tumor was benign - - no cancer at all. What a relief! But the nightmare had just begun.

Although she was in her early 50s, she was still having periods, not into menopause yet. The hysterectomy threw her into surgical menopause overnight. Previously, she had diabetes as well. Suddenly, her blood pressure went out of control, her cholesterol level shot up, and her headaches were almost unbearable. With all the hormones going out of whacky, she started HRT, (Hormone Replacement Therapy) which relieved her menopause symptoms and her high blood pressure was getting under control as well. But six months later, she was found to have early stage breast cancer, clearly triggered by the HRT, so she had to stop the treatment immediately. But the whacky again hormone level brought the hypertension back, worsened the diabetes, and the cholesterol level was out of balance again. But because of her body's sensitivity to breast cancer, she couldn't use HRT.

I am sure Sandra was not the only woman affected by HRT.

According to National Women's Health Network, the United States has the highest rate of hysterectomies in the industrialized world, and hysterectomy is the second-most frequently performed surgical procedure (after cesarean sections) for U.S. women. Approximately 600,000 hysterectomies are performed annually in the United States, and approximately *20 million American women* have had a hysterectomy.

Studies show that most hysterectomies performed in the United States are not medically necessary, evidenced by the fact that today, approximately 90 percent of hysterectomies are performed electively.

The National Women's Health Network (NWHN) believes that unnecessary hysterectomies have needlessly put women at risk, and that health care providers should recognize the value of a woman's reproductive organs beyond their reproductive capacity and search for alternatives before resorting to life-changing operations.

Quoted in the Los Angeles Times, NWHN Executive Director Cindy Pearson says, "I advise any woman who is not in a life-threatening situation to see someone else besides a surgeon to explore nonsurgical options first."

I strongly believe there are circumstances, such as malignant tumors or other medically required circumstances, where you may have to accept to completely or partially remove the affected organs in order to save your life. Otherwise I would encourage you to keep all your organs, especially your ovaries, from being surgically removed.

According to NWHN, a hysterectomy may be a medically necessary intervention in the case of several life-threatening conditions:

- Invasive cancer of the uterus, cervix, vagina, fallopian tubes, and/or ovaries
- Unmanageable infection
- Unmanageable bleeding

- Serious complications during childbirth, such as a rupture of the uterus

For other conditions, NWHN believes that it is advisable to evaluate all options before resorting to major surgery.

It is commonly known that western medicine considers the uterus no longer necessary or useful for women who no longer desire to have children, let alone for menopausal women. It is startling to me that western culture is conditioned to view our body as separate parts with no relationship or connection with one another.

Just think about what you see from ads: take this pill for insomnia, take that pill for headaches, another pill for stomach aches, drink this for fever, and use this nasal spray for a sinus condition...

Most of the time we don't really know how the body is interconnected and how each part of our body affects each other.

TCM believes the uterus still has value even for women who no longer desire to have children even though it produces lower levels of hormones. Our body is not an assemblage of isolated organs. All of them are interdependent and interrelated. Everything connects through Qi.

TCM's wisdom has been in existence for thousands of years; it applies the principal of Qi, yin and yang, and the five elements to guide you to live a life with quality and longevity. What you are learning from this book will give you the foundation to help you understand what created menopause symptoms in the first place, and what you can do about them so you can have a flourishing life for many years to come.

It is a very under-appreciated fact that the ovaries continue carrying impact and power in keeping our body in balance, even after menstrual periods completely stop. You should therefore be very cautious if you are faced with the drastic decision about having a hysterectomy involving ovary removal.

In my personal opinion, unless your condition is absolutely life-threatening, I would not elect for any surgery that would remove any organs. In most cases, our health issues can be reversed if we know their root cause, rather than just alleviating the symptoms. Understanding the root cause of any health issue leads us to find the right solution.

When my uterine fibroid grew to 10 cm, it required surgical intervention to remove it so my body would have the opportunity to recoup, recover, and rejuvenate. To have that tumor growing from 3 cm to 10 cm says a lot about my ignorance about my own body, and about how I ignored all the warning signs that my body showed me through all my menstrual problems and other health battles. I did not have the right information to decode what my body was trying to tell me about my situation. By the point when I knew I had to do something, it became a difficult choice between surgery or herbal remedies. It was a battle of getting a second chance for my body with newly equipped wisdom and knowledge to rebuild my health.

In certain cases, you may have to remove just the uterus while keeping the ovaries intact.

It is easy to fall into the trap that once you no longer want to have children, it is tempting to remove all the female organs to reduce worry about contracting uterine cancer, ovarian cancer, or other related ailments. Just because you no longer desire to have children, it does not follow that your female organs are no longer useful.

Long-term Risks of Hysterectomy

Removal of the uterus and ovaries in the early forties or even earlier may increase risks of heart attack, and (even when ovaries are not removed) chances of experiencing some other serious health issues.

Hysterectomies have also been associated with urinary problems, such as increased frequency, incontinence, fistula, and urinary tract infections; sexual function problems, such as decrease in sexual sensations and lack of lubrication; depression or psychological stress (stemming from feelings associated with losing reproductive organs); hormone deficiencies, which may be caused by removal of the ovaries, or a decrease in blood supply to the ovaries.

According to "Hysterectomy: a Collection of Women's Personal Experiences" by Elizabeth Ploude, it was noted that "the hysterectomized women who are most adversely affected are those who also had either one or both of their ovaries removed or had them compromised by the surgery, creating instant menopause. These women can suffer debilitating damage and many are not able to find the help they need to fully recover.

Their stories reveal the great disruption of ovary removal, or impairment of ovarian function, has on the rest of body, a disruption that has not been recognized or honored up to this point by mainstream doctors. Ovaries-removed women are the ones who suffer year in and year out, attempting to regain the health they had prior to surgery."

Ultimately, it is a situation-specific and individual-specific decision with regard to what kind of surgical intervention is best for you. I hope you can overcome any fear that you are facing and understand the pros and cons of each different scenario, and take into account the long-term impact on your life.

It can be scary. I was scared to death at the time, but I hope you are encouraged by my story and be brave enough to ask for what you want and make it happen, because you are the only one responsible for getting what you want and making your life better. Doctors will help you only if you know what you want.

The #4 Secret: You Will Have Smooth Menopause Without Suffering Any Menopausal Symptoms If You Start Listening to Your Body Today...

The best cure is prevention. Starting today, do not ignore any of your menstrual cycle problems, be it cramps, mood swings, spotting, early or delayed periods, extended periods, blood clots, etc.

Take a look at your lifestyle and your emotional state. Start to examine your life, and start some exercises in self-reflection.

Are you happy? If so, what makes you happy? Then do more things that make you happy. If not, why? What makes you unhappy? Try to reduce your exposure to things that make you unhappy.

Avoid blaming anyone else; avoid thinking other people caused your unhappiness, because ultimately, you are responsible for your own life. No one can make you happy unless you are happy yourself.

Not everyone has a difficult menopause, though the majority of women in western society experience menopause problems to some extent. You may wonder why this is happening to you.

I asked the same question myself about my earlier health struggles. I have been there and done that; now you don't have to go through it, because I can tell you why and you can see whether or not your body was out of balance long before your symptoms appeared.

I don't believe that we intentionally ignore all the warning signs that our body sends us; we simply do not have the right information to decode them.

It took me such exhausting and extensive research and relentless efforts to dig through more than 300 ancient TCM books to finally decipher the code of how and why I got all those health problems at the first place. With that knowledge today, eight years later, I am able to enjoy radiant health like never before.

So let me assure you that you are not alone. I have an MBA -- I am very well educated. I thought I knew a lot of things, yet I did not know my own body.

We live in a society that bombards us with information; most of the time we don't know what is right or wrong, which way we should follow. We try many things. We have a strong desire and willingness to improve our health, yet not everything is working. The confusing part is that most of the time we don't even have any clue what to believe and what not to believe.

My personal experience taught me that if something is working, your body knows. If you don't feel any difference from what you are trying, then obviously your body needs that fundamental boost of the acquired Qi to bring it back to its optimal state, so it will work following the law of nature, to heal itself, to rejuvenate itself, then something will happen, naturally and effortlessly.

Do not ignore the symptoms. If you can, please do not use pain killers for your headache, your migraine, or use ibuprofen for your menstrual cramps, or do not burn the lining of your uterus to stop spotting. Not only will the medication aggravate liver Qi stagnation even further, but also you lose the opportunity to give your body what it needs at the time it needs to prevent worse problems down the road. Temporary relief sometimes makes you feel good, but in the long run you are going to suffer more, much more. So be aware.

I encourage you to attentively listen to your body, to watch minor warning signs at an early stage, to do a reality check on your life, to be able to restore your body to its harmonious state sooner rather than later.

For any woman, if you are over 35 years old, it is in your best interests to be in tune to your body's peri-menopause signs. The quality of your menstrual period is the number one indicator of how healthy you are. Problems will first show during your period, so be in tune to your body and to your monthly cycle, then in the long term your quality of life and longevity will be tremendously improved.

Many of us have not taken very good care of ourselves, though we believe we have.

Before you turn 50, this is the last great opportunity for you to become truly healthy and address any problems you are having and prepare for the years ahead to be healthy and joyful.

Menopause is a real gateway that offers a chance for renewal of our bodies, minds and especially spirits. You can have a long happy vibrant journey without hormone therapy.

Even if you are currently suffering from menopause symptoms, chances are your body may have been out of balance for quite a while. If you already tried everything, but still don't feel any better, there is a solution. I am giving you secret recipes that you can easily brew at home. You can rest assured that your life will never be the same and you can heal yourself. Or if you are in peri-menopause, don't delay one single minute to get your radiant health back. You can save yourself a lot of struggle as you reach the age of menopause.

According to TCM theory, menopausal symptoms seem complicated, but essentially they result from a deficiency in "Yin." Yin is the energy of stillness, nighttime and coolness. Yin depletion can cause yang functions to become erratic and flare up, creating headaches, hot flashes, night sweats, vaginal and skin dryness, insomnia or irritability. In Asian cultures, Yin deficiency is commonly treated successfully with foods and herbs.

TCM has been effectively treating menopausal symptoms for thousands of years in China. I have read some studies published in western media discussing the connection of "Spleen Qi (Energy)" to a healthy reproductive system and well-balanced hormones, especially for women. "Spleen Qi" is the Master of the entire digestive system and determines how your entire body functions. Our ability to achieve our highest genetic potential is directly impacted by the foods we eat and the ways we handle stress in our environment. A strong "Spleen Qi" will enable your body to absorb the nutrients from what you eat and drink in an optimal way.

TCM always thinks about your health in terms of your Qi, which is the basis of the efficacy of all its treatments. TCM operates from the premise that as long as your Qi remains strong and flows freely and your body works in harmony, disease or illness cannot enter -- not even cancer. The opposite is true as well. If your Qi is weak and not flowing freely and your body's organs are not working in harmony, disease or illness can and do enter.

Western women, for the most part, have no idea that there is another way, a time-tested way that can change their whole lives. In China, women easily get great support from TCM through herbs and food. For thousands of years, millions of women have chosen this path and discovered a natural, healthy way to complete their life's journey. The time-tested nature of TCM should help reassure you of it efficacy and effectiveness.

TCM is a complete healing philosophy whose principles and theories have existed unaltered for thousands of years. Above all, it understands how to see, really see, and treat the whole person –body, mind, emotions, and spirit -- each of which must be carefully nurtured for lasting health and longevity.

You might be surprised that Chinese women are as perplexed about why American women don't understand what Yin deficiency means, just as American women are perplexed about why Chinese women rarely suffer menopausal symptoms.

As we age, we need to find an effective way to nurture our body, to replenish, nourish, and rejuvenate women's "Spleen Qi" energy, nourish kidney "Yin" deficiency and help bring our body back to its balanced and harmonious state, which is the fundamental for rebuilding our entire body and system to its optimal and balanced state.

The #5 Secret: Your Body's In-Born Power to Produce Female Hormones; Even after Menopause

Your body is designed to produce enough hormones for you to enjoy and sustain your longevity even after your periods come to an end. Even though it will not produce as much as in your child-bearing years, it should be sufficient for you to have a healthy and abundant life. You should never doubt it.

According to Heritage Notes from Fu Qing Zhu for Women, before your periods end, the liver is the most important hormone-regulating organ. *For gynecological problems, smoothing out and replenishing Liver Qi is the most effective solution*. For women to have radiant health, the best starting point is to regulate the menstrual period cycle to ensure it is smooth and problem- free.

This does not necessarily mean that after your menstrual periods end, you don't need to manage your stress or Liver Qi. The smoothness of Liver Qi is a direct reflection of your emotional state.

As we mentioned previously, Liver Qi very easily becomes stagnated if you have suppressed anger, depression, or any other emotional distress. Any Liver Qi stagnation will compromise the condition of other organs, and your body will start getting out of balance and out of harmony.

According to Heritage Notes from Fu Qing Zhu For Women, for women who already stopped the menstrual cycle, replenishing the Spleen Qi is the most effective way to bring health back on track. After your periods end, the Spleen is the most important organ regulating hormones.

According to TCM, your body is designed to produce healthy and abundant hormones even as you age. In order for your body to continue having that capability, you need to keep your Spleen Qi strong. The Spleen Qi is the master of entire digestive system and it determines how the entire body works in harmony.

Why is the digestive system so important?

Think of it this way. How does your body take nutrients other than utilizing the in-born finite Qi? It is from what you eat and drink. Our body's digestive system is very sophisticated. It takes everything you eat or drink and converts it into something to be used by your entire body. So you either nurture or deplete your body from what you eat and drink.

The reason is simple. If what you eat and drink does not provide necessary nutrients, or contains harmful materials such as excessive chemicals, artificial flavorings, or other damaging elements, your body has to work much harder to eliminate the toxins. This exhausts extra Qi, your finite life force. Over time, if you don't replenish the Qi, your body and your body's immune system will be in a compromised state, leaving your body vulnerable to disease. This is the reason that as we start aging, we start becoming vulnerable to a lot of epidemic diseases.

Now it is obvious that just eating healthy is not enough, and just maintaining a healthy life style is not enough either. If your Spleen Qi is weakened, be it from natural aging, or rapidly depleting from excessive use or sometimes abuse, you just don't feel good even you eat healthy. This is because your body is not taking everything you are eating and drinking and converting it into something essential to nurture your body efficiently.

Without continued nurturing and nourishing from what you eat and drink, your body will soon exhaust its in-born finite Qi and your body soon become vulnerable for all kinds of diseases. Therefore to effectively convert what you eat and drink to something to replenish and build your Qi reserve is crucial in maintaining your youth and health. No matter how magic a potion might be, if your digest system is not strong, your body will not benefit from it. This is the reason that in order to let your body heal, and in order to release your body's in-born rejuvenation power, to boost your spleen Qi is always the first thing that you want to do. With the strengthened spleen Qi, your body can take the healthy food you eat, and the supplement you take and convert them into the essential energy to nurture and replenish your body. It's interesting to notice that even the same food or supplements could have completely different impact to different people. The strength of the spleen Qi or the healthiness of the digestive system is the key for sustainable health and longevity.

According to TCM, a strong Spleen Qi also directly relates to how restfully you sleep. We all know cell repairs happen when you sleep. When you sleep better, your body rejuvenates better.

In order to treat any issues or problems, you need to boost the efficiency of your digestive system first, so your body can absorb all the nutrients from everything that your eat and drink. With continued effective nurturing, your body will acquire sufficient Qi to heal from any health issues and extend your longevity effortlessly.

The #6 Secret: You Don't Ever Need Hormone Replacement Therapy (HRT)

Risks of Hormone Replacement Therapy...

Hormone Replacement Therapy only provides temporary relief for your symptoms. In the long term, not only your health will be severely impacted and placed at risk by HRT, but your entire body, your body's natural in-born regulating and healing power will also be severely jeopardized.

If you take hormones, it will jeopardize your body's own power to produce them. Any drugs have side effects, which can further weaken your body's energy system. Your own internal Qi, which has already declined, will even get lazier and the longer you take the drugs, the less chance you have to heal yourself with its inborn capability, and the less chance you have to reactivate your body's ability to produce enough estrogen later on.

Furthermore, HRT carries many risks for potential side effects, particularly breast cancer and uterine cancer. When used alone, ERT estrogen has been shown to increase the risk of endometrial cancer by 400 to 800 percent. Furthermore, the risk of cancer increases with prolonged use of estrogen.

Dilemma: HRT or No HRT

When menopausal symptoms become unbearable, most doctors in Western medicine would suggest using hormone replacement therapy to replenish the shortage of hormone in the body. Most women are reluctant to use HRT, yet they have fear about what might happen if they do not use HRT. The fact is that you are pretty much left on your own to figure out what to do if you don't want to use HRT.

Most western women lack the access to the knowledge that there is another way, a time-tested way that can change their whole life, a powerful natural method to effectively treat the root cause of menopause.

If you take hormones, your own power to produce from within is diminished. Drugs weaken the body's energy system. Qi gets lazy, and the longer you take them the less chance you have to heal yourself, to reactivate your ability to produce enough during later years. If you do take the opportunity to become balanced during menopause transitional time, you can reach a new level of health. If you are healthy your body can heal itself from practically anything.

Now back to the difference between Western and Eastern medicine. In Western medicine, the main cause of menopausal symptoms is seen as a lack of estrogen and progesterone production. However, just because something is lacking, does not necessarily mean that replacing it will restore the normal function to complex organs. What is lacking occurred as a result of a number of interrelated and interdependent physical, spiritual, and emotional changes.

When you were young, why you did not have a problem? What has changed? Is it possible this condition can be fixed from inside? Will HRT fix the root cause of the problem? How long should you be on HRT? What happens if you stop it?

Treatment involves increasing the acquired Qi to make it strong and flowing smoothly without any stagnation or blockage, so that your body can work in harmony.

I am a perfect example. Eight years later, not only I am healthier than before, but my periods and hormones are more balanced than ever. I did not achieve this overnight. Along the past years, I had some period problems here and there. I not only paid very close attention to my period, I also diligently identified the root causes for throwing me into such whacky episodes. What specific event, what kind of pressure and stress from where, those were the questions I asked myself often. Then I put into immediate action to manage stress and my emotional state, thus to restore my health. With equipped knowledge and wisdom, it became easier and easier to recognize the small disturbance to my health and never gave it chance to ever show in larger scale.

Estrogen production is related to healthy kidney Qi and to a certain extent with other organs, especially the liver. In order for your body to produce adequate hormones, each of these organs needs to function properly and communicate harmoniously with one another. It is vital to maintain the connection back and forth.

As you age, Qi declines and organs gradually lose the ability to work in harmony. The ability of your body to function diminishes, or stops entirely at some point. When this is reversed your body will capitalize on its natural ability to once again produce hormones to regulate your body in harmony. Even at lower levels, it will be enough to maintain your health.

Think about the millions of women who went through menopause before HRT was invented. It definitely would not make any sense that your body was created without the capability necessary to survive without external intervention. Your body is part of the nature that God creates. God already created a way for you to continue flourishing only if you have been responsible, providing your body what it needs, and your body will work in nature's way to defeat everything and keep you in radiant health.

Studies and Statistics from National Cancer Institute about HRT

The U.S. Food and Drug Administration currently advise women to use HRT for the shortest time and at the lowest dose possible to control the symptoms of menopause.

According to a study conducted by Women's Health Initiative (WHI) and published by National Cancer Institute, although Menopause Hormone Therapy (MHT) provides short-term benefits, such as relief from hot flashes and vaginal dryness, a number of health concerns are associated with its use, including increased risk for certain cancers.

Research from the WHI has shown that MHT is associated with the following ailments:

- **Urinary incontinence**. Use of estrogen plus progestin increased the risk of urinary incontinence.
- **Dementia**. Use of estrogen plus progestin doubled the risk of developing dementia among postmenopausal women age 65 and older.
- **Stroke, blood clots, and heart attack**. Women who took either combined hormone therapy or estrogen alone had an increased risk of stroke, blood clots, and heart attack.

For women in both groups, however, this risk returned to normal levels after they stopped taking the medication.

- **Breast cancer**. Women who took estrogen plus progestin were more likely to be diagnosed with breast cancer. The breast cancers in these women were larger and more likely to have spread to the lymph nodes by the time they were diagnosed. The number of breast cancers in this group of women increased with the length of time that they took the hormones and decreased after they stopped taking the hormones.

These studies also showed that both combination and estrogen-only hormone use made mammography less effective for early detection of breast cancer. Women taking hormones had more repeat mammograms to check on abnormalities and more breast biopsies to determine whether abnormalities were cancerous.

According to Cancer Statistics Review referenced in Harvard Women's Health Watch, women who have been receiving HRT or ERT (Estrogen Replacement Therapy) for five years or more have an overall 305 percent greater risk of breast cancer than those who have not. When used alone, as in ERT, estrogen has been shown to increase the risk of endometrial cancer by 400 to 800 percent.

The risk of cancer increases with prolonged use of estrogen, and with age.

Ironically, in order to acquire whatever protection estrogen may offer from heart disease and osteoporosis, you must pass through the risk phase of breast cancer and keep taking these drugs.

- Lung cancer. Women who took combined hormone therapy had the same risk of lung cancer as women who took the placebo. However, among those who were diagnosed with lung cancer, women who took estrogen plus progestin were more likely to die of the disease than those who took the placebo.
- Colorectal cancer. In the initial study report, women taking combined hormone therapy had a lower risk of colorectal cancer than women who took the placebo. However, the colorectal tumors that arose in the combined hormone therapy group were more advanced at detection than those in the placebo group. There was no difference in either the risk of colorectal cancer or the stage of disease at diagnosis between women who took estrogen alone and those who took the placebo.

The #7 Secret: The Myth about the Three Biggest Postmenopausal Health Problems, and How to Take Preventive Steps to Avoid Them

Heart disease, breast cancer and osteoporosis are the three major health problems that women fear most as they go through menopause, because these three diseases are the most life-threatening for women, especially post- menopause.

Heart Disease

According to published statistics from the Center for Disease Control, heart disease is the number one cause of death in the U.S., also the number one killer of women, accounting for half of all deaths of women over the age of 50.

In TCM's perspective, whenever the heart has a problem, unless it is related to a birth defect or genetically inherited deficiency, it is typically the result of a disrupted relationship of the heart with other organs. As we mentioned in the TCM principles and holistic view of the body, a heart problem is not just in the heart alone, so the treatment should involve treating its related organs: in most cases it is the kidney Qi that controls it, or the Spleen Qi.

Kidney Qi naturally declines with age, and most people tend to have Kidney Qi deficiency as they get older. Specifically for heart problems related to post menopause, TCM believes the root cause is severe Kidney Yin and Spleen Qi deficiency.

Symptoms of poor heart function often appear after menopause, including palpitations, other abnormal cardiac rhythms, insomnia, and high blood pressure. So, if a woman has been generally healthy without any obvious cardiovascular problems before menopause, and the heart problems only start appearing afterwards, it is likely that the heart problem is directly related to the root cause of menopause, the Kidney Qi deficiency and weakened Spleen Qi.

As we have emphasized in previous chapters, we were all born with finite in-born Qi. As this in-born Qi declines as we age, unless we replenish it, our body naturally weakens. All the organs start functioning in a compromised state, causing our body to function in a disharmonized state.

In modern society, our hit-or-miss diets, chaotic schedules, and hectic lifestyle all accelerate the imbalance of our body. So before the natural aging process even starts, our body has already run out of balance, exhausting our in-born Qi prematurely. This is the reason that the average age of a lot of medical issues happens much sooner than we anticipate. There are women going through menopause before they turn 45. This is not normal. We should not accept this as such.

By simply replenishing your Kidney Qi and boosting your Spleen Qi, you are not only curing medical issues but preventing them from getting worse. If a woman can increase her Kidney Qi effectively, and learn the proper way to take care of herself, she will be less likely to suffer from serious heart problems as she ages.

In the oldest TCM philosophies, there were two very popular schools regarding which should be replenished first in fighting against aging or pre-mature aging.

One school believed that replenishing Kidney Yin is the first step to regulate the body's natural power to rejuvenate. Once Kidney Yin is plentiful and abundant, your hair, your libido, and your sexual drive will all come alive. Then the abundant Yin will further nourish all the other organs to bring them back to a harmonious state.

Another school believes that replenishing and strengthening

Spleen Qi is the fundamental way to heal and fight any aging signs, as all the organs depend on the essence converted from what you eat and drink. Without strengthened Spleen Qi, all other efforts will be compromised.

In my personal healing journey and all the years that I have been maintaining radiant health, I think that to boost, to replenish and to strengthen our Spleen Qi is essential and fundamental for everything else and beyond. Our Spleen Qi oversees the entire digestive system and how the body functions. "Without digestion functioning well, without spleen Qi, you have no life, you are dead."

Again, the theory is quite simple: everything you are trying to do with your body have to start with what you eat and drink.

We already know just eating healthy is not enough, because if your body is not absorbing 100% of what you eat or drink, no matter how healthy your diet or life style, the result will be minimal.

Once you strengthen your Spleen Qi, your body is going to function like a newly overhauled machine. It's like giving your body a second chance from a brand new starting point. Nothing is more exciting than that!

Why is it so important to strengthen the Spleen Qi and the digestive system?

If you don't have strong Qi, no matter what herbal concoction you are trying, your body will not be able to absorb it. Your body cannot take the essence from what you eat and drink.

Not everyone was born equal, and not everything works the same way for everyone either. Foods, drugs, tonics, vitamins, minerals, supplements, energy boosters, etc. work better for some and less well for others. The secret is that without addressing the root cause of your hormone imbalance, even if you eat healthy or exercise regularly, all of your efforts will not be maximized.

Osteoporosis

Osteoporosis affects at least 25% of Caucasian American women. It is another major health problem in this country. It afflicts more than 10 million Americans, 80% of whom are post-menopausal women.

Each year, osteoporosis causes an estimated 1.5 million bone fractures including 350,000 hip fractures. Seventy percent of those suffering from osteoporosis do not return to previous pre-injury status.

According to Western Medicine, Osteoporosis is a widespread metabolic bone disease characterized by decreased bone mass and poor bone quality. It leads to an increased frequency in fractures of the hip, spine, and wrist.

According to Traditional Chinese Medicine, bones are tissues of the Kidney Qi and get their nourishment for growth of new bone tissue from strong or strengthened Kidney Qi. TCM believes that bone problems can be relieved indirectly through replenishing and strengthening the Kidney Qi.

Let's say you break your wrist at work, or injure your knees while playing sports. In order to speed recovery which requires promoting the new bone tissue growth, TCM doctors will prescribe a formulation that replenishes and strengthens the Kidney Qi and Spleen Qi.

When you are young, your body will heal from those bone fractures or injuries much more easily than when you are older.

As you age, bone problems seem to get worse and worse. Why? Think about another example. As we age, we start losing our teeth, and then we feel our knees are no longer as strong ...

As we mentioned previously, your Kidney Qi declines naturally as you age, so the aging process can be prevented and reversed through replenishing the Kidney Qi; when the Kidney Qi is strengthened, your bone tissue growth will be improved significantly as well.

Yes, aging is a natural process, but we can slow down the aging curve and we can extend longevity through replenishing Kidney Qi and strengthening Spleen Qi.

Ultimately, it all boils down to the one fundamental principal to replenish your body with what it needs and follow the law of nature, and everything else will take care of itself.

I cannot emphasize enough how important it is for you to be in tune with your body and how important it is for you to take preventative steps to start nourishing your body as early as you can, to avoid serious problems from ever appearing. The best way to treat osteoporosis is to address its root cause, and understand the value of prevention. TCM's approach in treating osteoporosis focuses on two main objectives: one is to replenish Kidney Yin Deficiency and the other is to strengthen the Spleen Qi, which controls the digestive system.

As you age, you spend your Qi much faster than you rejuvenate it, which means that over time, your body will be out of balance. When you spend more than you generate, you know for sure that is not sustainable. So how do you achieve longevity? The answer is simple: ensure that you exhaust your Qi less than you generate, or conserve more and replenish more while you spend less

That is why just taking calcium supplements is not going to help you much to avoid osteoporosis. Science has already proven that mineral nutrients do not work as we think; if you take calcium, then your body will have enough calcium. Calcium needs to work with other minerals together in a highly sophisticated way to be absorbed and processed by your body. If the organ responsible for processing the absorption and delivering the essence is not working efficiently, chances are you will get little or no benefit from taking the supplement.

Supplements work for some people more efficiently than for others. As we mentioned previously, not everyone is born equally with regard to physical attributes, health, and strength of our in-born Qi; certain people absorb nutrients more efficiently than other people. You need very strong digestion to efficiently and effectively extract the essence from food, herbs, tonics, and supplements.

Sooner or later, everyone develops some degree of bone loss. It is nature's way. We all wish our bones could stay as strong as they were in our 20s, but the reality is that is it not possible. But it is possible to continue replenishing and nourishing your body properly so you can slow down the rate at which your bone loss occurs.

Even if you are currently suffering from osteoporosis, by simply adding classic herbs to your diet or even drinking nourishing potions from TCM herbs, you can re-build your body to a better state so it can fight aging and even reverse its effects.

The best way is to let your body follow nature's way, so that your body will truly become part of this universe and achieve longevity.

Breast Cancer

Breast Cancer in the United States - In the U.S. breast cancer is the second-most frequently diagnosed cancer for women.

According to Breast Cancer Facts & Figures published by the American Cancer Society, in 2013, an estimated 232,340 new cases of invasive breast cancer were diagnosed among women, as well as an estimated 64,640 additional cases of DCIS (in situ) breast cancer.

> *"Ductal carcinoma in situ (DCIS) is the most common type of non-invasive breast cancer. Ductal means that the cancer starts inside the milk ducts, carcinoma refers to any cancer that begins in the skin or other tissues (including breast tissue) that cover or line the internal organs, and in situ means "in its original place." DCIS is called "non-invasive" because it hasn't spread beyond the milk duct into any normal surrounding breast tissue. DCIS isn't life-threatening, but having DCIS can increase the risk of developing an invasive breast cancer later on."*
>
> – Quoted from
> BreastCancer.org

Excluding cancers of the skin, breast cancer is the most common cancer among U.S. women, accounting for 29% of newly diagnosed cancers. The total number of deaths from breast cancer for women is second only to lung cancer.

Breast cancer incidence and death rates generally increase with age: 79% of new cases and 88% of breast cancer deaths occurred in women 50 years of age and older.

During 2006-2010, the median age at the time of breast cancer diagnosis was 61.14. This means that half the women who developed breast cancer were 61 years of age or younger at the time of diagnosis.

A woman living in the US has a 12.3%, or a 1 in 8, lifetime risk of being diagnosed with breast cancer compared to that of 1 in 11 in the 1970s.

TCM's View of Breast Cancer

In ancient TCM books, breast cancer was described as a hard node inside a woman's breast caused by extended and prolonged periods of her unhappiness, and the long-term depression that suppressed the Liver Qi flow.

In TCM's view, the root cause of breast cancer is Kidney Qi

deficiency and poor Liver Qi function. The reason is that TCM believes that the kidney controls a broad complex of the endocrine and immune system. The liver controls the stomach, whose meridian passes through the breasts.

Liver Qi is very sensitive to any emotional turmoil. For women, any suppressed anger, extended period of stress from any aspect of life will have a deep impact to liver Qi's free and smooth flow, thus planting the seed for a later developed mass, tumor or cancer.

TCM believes that most cancers, except those caused by sudden drastic external environment changes, such as nuclear exposure, poison, birth defect, etc. are attributed to Qi stagnation, be it liver Qi, Spleen Qi, Stomach Qi, etc.

There is an ancient TCM saying, "Where there is Qi blockage, there is a disease, mass or tumor; where Qi flows freely and smoothly, disease has nowhere to enter, let alone a mass or tumor."

TCM also believes that it takes between four and forty years for cancer to develop. So if you are diagnosed with cancer, it is likely that your body has been out of balance for years.

Breast cancer, like any disease, starts first as Qi stagnation or deficiency. From this point on, your lifestyle determines whether or not this stagnant condition will progress to a mass or turn into something cancerous.

When women complain of vague, intermittent discomforts that rarely show on scientific tests, they are really speaking in the language of Qi. You may experience occasional breast tenderness. You may periodically have headaches. When you rest they seem to go away. You may take pain pills or aspirin to relieve those symptoms. In the Western world, we are conditioned to believe that these are minor, insignificant events. They are actually not!

When the body is healthy, it does not have physical, mental or emotional problems. Any minor complaints like the ones we just mentioned are the first signs to tell you that your body is out of balance of Qi. You need to pay attention to them before they become much bigger.

In modern society, we have been conditioned to be tough, to work like men, to not complain about minor discomforts. We have never been taught to listen closely to our body, to carefully watch for early warning signs. The truth is that if a functional disorder continues unchecked because there are occasional minor events, physical evidence of it will eventually appear.

For example, a woman might begin to experience menstrual problems, PMS, breast tenderness, migraines, mood swings and more. Without being watched or treated, these symptoms can worsen over time and develop into other serious gynecological problems, or may even lead to a mass or tumor.

If the mass or tumor develops and is combined with other internal and external problems, it can easily turn into cancer.

If your Qi has been strong enough and your organs function in harmony, the cancer will never have the chance to progress. The appearance of cancer is the ultimate evidence that your body's weakened Qi is not able to suppress the progression of a mass or tumor from accelerating.

Thousands of years ago, TCM already identified the root cause of cancer as being Qi stagnation and blockage from either internal or external factors.

American Cancer Society's statement in its Cancer Facts & Figures still says that knowledge about the risk factors to prevent breast cancer have not been translated into practical ways to prevent it.

If you do not have breast cancer, the best way to prevent it is to focus on strengthening your Qi, ensuring your Liver Qi flows smoothly and boosting your Spleen Qi so that your body will defend itself against further progression of any disease. Cancer will never even have a chance, if you do this diligently.

To have a strong Spleen Qi is the most fundamental condition for achieving health and longevity so you can continue enjoying the abundance that life offers.

Conclusion

Having read this far, you have already gained rich understanding that you do have the opportunity to regain your heath if you start taking action today to be in charge of your own health and your own body. It is never too late to start.

So begin today and be more in tune to all the sometimes subtle warning signs show up in your body; whether it is period abnormalities, headaches or insomnia. Do not try to mask any discomfort using pain killers. Do not use sleeping pills to solve your insomnia.

Also, be aware of your stress levels and develop your own ways to manage your stress and your emotional state.

Start doing more things that make you happy. Ultimately the happiness comes from within, the inside of you rather than being validated by any external factors.

When you face a decision for any surgery related to your reproductive organs, take an active role in fully evaluating the pros and cons of the surgery.

Make your best efforts to preserve your organs whenever the technology and the doctors' skill allow. Do not be afraid of the hassles that you may have to deal with in the process. It is your body and you do have the responsibility of giving your body the best chance to recover with its full potential and capability intact.

Believe in yourself and the power of your body. God gives us the amazing self-healing power to defeat any diseases. You can unleash that power to allow your body to heal, and rejuvenate in the natural way.

Be brave to allow yourself to live a life with symptom-free menopause, and you can do it with the time tested remedies that I am attaching at the end of this book. Once you learn how to nourish and nurture your body in the way that it was intended and originally designed, you will be amazed by how effortless the healing and self-rejuvenating starts taking place.

Have faith and be grateful. The best part of your life has just begun....

Small Ways You Can Start Today to Transform Your Life Forever

1. <u>Drink a glass of warm water first thing in the morning</u>

In the morning after you wake up, the first thing you should do is to drink a glass (at least 10 oz.) of warm water, a little bit warmer than lukewarm.

To maximize the benefit, you can also either add one teaspoon of apple cider vinegar or a teaspoon of freshly squeezed lemon juice with a tablespoon of honey to adjust the taste. This gently warms up the spleen and awakens the digestive and kidney systems and helps cleanse all the wastes that the body metabolized and processed overnight.

Adding apple cider vinegar helps regulate the body's pH to create a more balanced inner environment to improve energy flow. It is also proven to help maintain healthy digestion.

Adding fresh lemon juice will help regulate and maintain your body's pH environment to alkaline. Numerous studies have proven that an alkaline environment will suppress the cancer cell growth in your body. If you have diligently maintained your body's pH to slightly alkaline, the chance for cancer growth is minimal to none.

Why honey? In Traditional Chinese Medicine, honey is a great nutritious food with essential micronutrients such as vitamins, iron, calcium and copper and key enzymes that help relieve heat, clear away toxins relieve pain and combat dehydration. It also helps nourish the energy (Yin) and strengthens the body's spleen, sharpens eyesight and brings out healthy, rosy cheeks. By simply taking a tablespoon every morning, honey can help prevent constipation as well.

Additional tip: if you are suffering from allergies, substitute commercially-available honey with local, unprocessed honey. It will work wonders in helping to relieve allergy symptoms.

When eating out, start with a cup of hot water with a few slices of lemon in it. This will ready the stomach for the food intake. Slowly incorporate drinking warm water in your daily routine. Try it first thing when you wake up in the morning, before you eat, and between your daily activities. Do this for a week and experience the health benefits. You will likely see some changes in your digestion, mood and energy levels. You can also see improvements from many chronic problems that you may be dealing with, like a decrease in menstrual pain or alleviation from mood swings or anxiety.

2. Reduce cold drink intake whenever possible.

Especially for women, drinking warm fluids all the time carries tremendous benefits to your Spleen Qi. The strength of your Spleen Qi is directly related to the length of your period.
If you have irregular bleeding or spotting for sure you want to strengthen your Spleen Qi first. With strong Spleen Qi, the spotting or irregular bleeding problem will go away by itself.

If you have difficulty losing weight, very likely your Spleen Qi is wet. The wet Spleen Qi will severely compromise your weight loss efforts. To simply reduce the cold drink intake and start drinking warm water the first thing in the morning when you wake up will help you easily shed a few pounds.

America prefers to drink cool or ice-cold water. This is mainly brought about by the early introduction of and adaption to refrigeration in the U.S. Cold beverages make Americans feel more refreshed—like drinking ice-cold beer or soda on a hot summer day. In other parts of the world, especially in China, drinking hot or warm beverages is the norm, mainly because of the associated health benefits.

According to Traditional Chinese Medicine, warmth is the most important thing dictating all physiological functions in our body. This warmth is called *Qi*. The Spleen Qi is the most important since it manifests how our entire body functions. Once your stomach receives food, it is the Spleen Qi that starts to transform the essence of that food into useful energy. When we constantly drink iced or refrigerated fluids, the cold causes your Spleen Qi to slow down and harden, creating the basis for pain and chronic diseases to develop. While these symptoms do not manifest immediately, they develop over time initially affecting our metabolism and digestion before spreading to other organs. These block the meridian channels, slow down blood circulation, and compromise organ functions to less than optimal ability.

Our body organs cannot immediately metabolize fluids that are below 37 degrees Celsius, the core body temperature, including 22 degree room temperature water. So the body is forced to work harder, wasting energy in order to make cold drinks warm enough for the body to use. This energy could have been better spent on healing illness, increasing immunity, etc.

Your body gets all of its energy and nutrition from the process that begins in the spleen and stomach. It is crucial to keep the

Spleen Qi energy flowing smoothly and drinking warm water and/or beverages will help ensure that.

3. **Fitness tip: Never consume cold drinks immediately after exercise.**

Drinking cold water immediately after exercise tends to shock the organs, and does not aid in helping the body too properly and naturally cool down.

This is because during exercise, internal body heat moves to the surface, causing sweating and hot exterior sensations, while in fact the interior has become cooler. So drinking a cold beverage aggravates the already-cold interior. Drinking warm water will help body's surface cool down naturally.

When you work out, let your sweat out naturally. Do not suppress your sweat by directly facing a fan or having a fan running on high in the room. This will suppress the benefits of working out and shut down your body when it is trying to eliminate all the toxins or excessive adrenaline.

You want to maximize the benefit from everything you do. Working out is a great way to relieve stress and get your body's metabolism running, and eliminate excessive hormones and toxins. Anything that suppresses that benefit carries potential harm to your body, though you may not always know or associate certain habits with your problems. It takes both knowledge and an open mind to ensure you are doing things appropriate to your body and not just the instant gratification from facing a fan or from drinking a chilled beverage.

A morning stretch, even just three or four minutes, produces tremendous benefits. It will warm up your body and eliminate soreness from sleep and keep your body Qi flowing and blood circulation in the optimal way.

Evening relaxation will help calm down your body, prepare it for deep sleep to effectively and efficiently rejuvenate and repair cell damage from the day.

4.   Pay close attention to your sleeping patterns.

Do not ever use sleeping pills if you don't have to. If you don't feel any harm from sleeping pills, that is likely because it simply hasn't manifested itself yet. By the time the harm of sleeping pill starts to show it will be too late to correct. Then your body will have to work much harder and may not be able to reverse the damage.

Pay close attention when you start having a hard time going to sleep or when you start waking up in the middle of the night and have a hard time going back to sleep; all these are signs that your body is functioning out of harmony and balance, especially signaling the weakening of your Spleen Qi.

If this is the case, take a moment to have some self-reflection to examine external factors that have possibly contributed to your physical state: stress from work, from life, from your spouse, from finances, from children. Meditate and solve the root cause to regain peace of mind, be grateful for everything you have, count your blessings, come up with active solutions to relieve the stress factors and regain your happiness.

For women, the best gift you can give to yourself is to be happy, no matter what, with strong inner peace, self-awareness, and self-control about your emotional state in any situation.

When a woman cannot sleep, it is just the beginning of a downward spiral. So be careful, very careful, when you start having sleep issues. Do not mask your sleeping problem with a pill. It can be used as temporary relief, but you need to look into your situation to address the root cause of what actually made your sleep pattern out of balance.

These things all seem small, but once you start implementing them little by little on a consistent basis, you will be amazed how easily and effortlessly your life can be transformed. If you just follow nature's way, then nature will take care of itself.

Simple and Classic TCM Formulas for Women to Enjoy Radiant Health at All Ages

This formula is named as Free Flow and Easy Wanderer Formula. It is the most classic and widely used formula in TCM for regulating women's hormones and promoting lasting health.

This classic formula can be used over the long term to have lifelong impact on women. It helps relieve Liver stagnation, replenish Spleen Qi and Kidney Yin. Especially for women, this formula will build and tone blood circulation as well.

As we mentioned previously, the liver is the most important organ for women in regulating overall hormone balance. The liver is also the most sensitive organ to any emotional distress. It is almost impossible for women not to have any emotional stress at all. Emotion is women's best friend, but it can be our worst enemy if we have no wisdom and knowledge to manage it well.

I would encourage you to constantly pay attention to your emotional state and your body's minor discomforts: your period, sleep patterns, your mood, etc... If you feel stressed out and feel your body out of balance and harmony, this formula will come in very handy and give you the most effective help at the time you need the most.

There are a total of six herbs in this formula:

Bupleurum Root:

Other Names: Honey root

Latin Name: Radix bupleuri

Chinese Pinxin Pronunciation: Chai Hu

Effects:

- o Smooth liver function, relieve liver Qi stagnation
- o Promote the flow of Qi, reduce internal heat
- o Regulate menstrual irregularities

Angelica root

Other Names: Dong Quai, or Tangkuei Root

Latin name: Radix Angelicae sinensis

Chinese Pinxin pronunciation: Dang Gui

Effects:

- o Tone and build blood, increase circulation
- o Regulate irregular menstruation
- o Replenish blood deficiency
- o Relieve pain due to internal blood and Qi stagnation

White Peony

Other Names: none

Latin Name: Radix Paeoniae Alba

Chinese Pinxin Pronounciation: Bai Shao Yao

Effects:

- o Nourish the blood
- o Regulate menstruation
- o Nourish the liver, balance liver function
- o Reinforce Yin Qi, stop irregular bleeding

Hoelen:

Other Names: Poria Mushroom

Latin Name: Poria (hoelen)

Chinese Pinxin Pronounciation: Bai Fu Ling

Effects:

- o Tone Spleen
- o Rid excess dampness of body
- o Tranquilize the spirit
- o Regulate and optimize body's metabolism

Chinese Licorice

Latin Name: Radix Glycyrrhizin

Chinese Pinxin Pronunciation: Gan Cao

Effects:

- o Increase Qi and overall vitality

- Tone Spleen function
- Relieve body internal heat
- Detoxify
- Harmonize the properties of other herbs in the formula

White Atraclylodes Rhizome:

Latin Name: Rhizoma Atractylodis Macrocephalae.

Chinese Pinxin Pronunciation: BaiZhu.

Effects:

- Strengthen the spleen and stomach
- Excrete dampness, especially from low abdominal area
- Relieve any digestive problem.

BaiZhu is the most classic herb in TCM to invigorate the Spleen Qi and Stomach Qi, remove dampness and activate the Spleen. It is very effective in boosting and strengthening the Spleen Qi and stomach Qi and water retention.

Function of the Formula

As we mentioned previously, to maintain a strong Spleen Qi directly determines how your stomach absorbs the essence and nutrients from what you eat and drink. Sufficient Spleen Qi and Stomach Qi also help protect the body from diseases.

Three of the herbs (Bupleurum, tang-kuei, and peony) are aimed at improving liver function, three (hoelen, atractylodes, baked licorice) are aimed at improving spleen function.

From another perspective: three of the herbs serve primarily as nourishing tonics (tang-kuei, peony, and baked licorice) and three serve primarily as herbs to alleviate stagnation (bupleurum, hoelen, and atractylodes).

The broad applications listed for *this Free Flow and Wanderer (Chinese pronouncing Xiao Yao San)* can be understood in terms of its objective: treating a fundamental underlying disorder, which is the obstructed flow of Qi that results from certain mental processes. The mind that has not learned how to face problems effectively, that struggles, strives, and competes, will cause the body's Qi to stagnate, which, over time, yields various symptoms and diseases.

The solution on the mental level is to be aware, understand, and meditate; on the physical level, the solution is to gently promote the smooth circulation of Qi.

This simple formula embodies the holistic principles of tonifying and dispersing in a balanced manner. The herbs benefit spleen and the liver, which are the two organs that are commonly involved in disharmony of Qi circulation.

I have since developed this pre-mixed formula from hand-selected, high quality ingredients. Each element is finely milled first to ensure the healing properties of the herbs will be completely extracted. Then, the tonic formula for each one-day serving is precisely mixed, blended and packed into a convenient pouch that's simple to use. I suggest you brew the tonic with our specially designed Empress' Secret thermos. This thermos will retain the temperature of the hot water long enough to release all the healing properties and flavor from the pre-mixed tonic formula. You can also use other high quality thermos, if you have one that performs well.

All that you need to do is fill the thermos with boiling water at night before you go to bed, then place the pouch in the thermos and let it brew overnight. The next morning when you get up, you will have this treasured, freshly brewed and delicious health tonic ready for you to drink. You can also take the thermos with you to enjoy it throughout the day. I can assure you that your life will never be the same if you stick to this regimen, and allow the tonic to naturally replenish and rejuvenate your body. Please visit my website: www.TheEmpressSecret.com for more information about this new product. It will soon be available in the online store.

The general rule of thumb is to drink this tonic for 5-7 days when you have noticeable discomfort before or during the period and noticeable period abnormalities, such as blood clots, ahead of schedule or delayed period, excessive bleeding or extended period, etc.

I have personally benefited tremendously from this formula. As women, rarely do we not have any emotional frustration, be it from work or life...we don't want stress, we try to avoid stress in our lives, but most times it is easier to say than to do.

This formula will become handy for you to not only replenish your body's blood and Qi, but also help soothe the liver stagnation that could potentially cause much worse health issues later stage. It will help relieve some obvious irregularities from our period so effectively. Even you do not have any obvious period irregularities; it is still very good for regulating your hormone balance, build blood and replenish your body.

Remember, the best cure is prevention. My personal journey has proved that this formula is the most precious self-help you can get and the best gift you can give to yourselves to maintain your radiant health.

I would strongly recommend any women at any age to drink this potion every 3-4 month for about 5-7 days; you will save yourself so much trouble from ever deteriorating health.

It is always better to start when you do not yet have any obvious symptoms. Even if you do notice discomfort here and there, it will help bring all organs in your body to a harmonious and balanced state to prevent further health issues even coming up.

The Wonder Formula for Women Currently Suffering from Menopause Symptoms

If you have read this far, I am sure you have already gained a holistic perspective about menopause, what caused that and why you are having menopause symptoms. Likely your body has been out of harmony for a while.

The first step you want to do is to examine your life style and your diet to make sure you eat healthy and live a balanced lifestyle.

This is very important. No matter how effective the potion, ultimately it is your healthy lifestyle that sustains your longevity and quality of life.

The next step is to have all your menopausal symptoms under control through boosting your fundamental Qi and replenishing your body with replenished Qi effectively.

Once your menopausal symptoms are under control, you can continue to replenish and nourish your body with acquired Qi to build sufficient Qi bank in your body. Then from there, you will either start, or continue or maintain your healthy lifestyle.

Healthy lifestyle is not just limited to eating healthy. You need to have a regular workout routine to keep the flexibility of your body. Also you want to have routine meditation or to develop your own way of dealing with the unexpected stress factors in your life.

The three basic herb ingredients that help to build body's fundamental Qi very effectively is abbreviated as "Shen, Ghi, Shu" -- Shen refers to Condonopsis, Ghi refers to Astragalus Root and Shu refers to BaiZhu.

Condonopsis Root:

Latin Name: Radix Codonopsis pilosulae

Chinese Pinxin pronunciation: Dang Shen

Effects:

- Tone the spleen and lung
- Promote and build blood and body fluids
- Increase Qi, especially Spleen Qi
- Promote sound sleep, relieve insomnia

Astragalus:

Latin Name: Radix Astragali seu Hedysari

Chinese Pinyin pronunciation: Huang Qi

Effects:

- Tone and boost body's Qi
- Boost immune system.
- Detoxify
- Replenish Qi deficiency and vital energy due to weakened body system from aging or chronic disease.
- Help strengthen Spleen function problems as well.

White Atraclylodes Rhizome:

Latin Name: Rhizoma Atractylodis Macrocephalae.

Chinese Pinxin Pronunciation: BaiZhu.

Effects:

- Strengthen the spleen and stomach
- Excrete dampness, especially from low abdominal area
- Help any digestive problem.

Bai Zhu is also one of the ingredients in Free Flow and Wanderer Formula. It further proves that the importance of Bai Zhu in regulating, boosting and rejuvenating the Spleen Qi function. With strengthened Spleen Qi, your body will start working wonders, following the law of nature to heal and to rejuvenate in the most natural way.

In order to relieve menopausal symptoms and to gradually eliminate HRT, you need to have these three ingredients as the very basic fundamental herbs, and then combine it with the formula of Free Flow and Wanderer.

If you are currently taking HRT and trying to get rid of HRT, start with this formula for at least 7-10 days. Start reducing the HRT dosages, cut pill in half or extend patch half times longer than normal use. Gradually reduce HRT until your body functions normally without it.

I have since developed this pre-mixed formula from hand-selected, high quality ingredients. Each element is finely milled first to ensure the healing properties of the herbs will be completely extracted. Then, the tonic formula for each one-day serving is precisely mixed, blended and packed into a convenient pouch that's simple to use. I suggest you brew the tonic with our specially designed Empress' Secret thermos. This thermos will retain the temperature of the hot water long enough to release all the healing properties and flavor from the pre-mixed tonic formula. You can also use other high quality thermos, if you have one that performs well.

All that you need to do is fill the thermos with boiling water at night before you go to bed, then place the pouch in the thermos and let it brew overnight. The next morning when you get up, you will have this treasured, freshly brewed and delicious health tonic ready for you to drink. You can also take the thermos with you to enjoy it throughout the day. I can assure you that your life will never be the same if you stick to this regimen, and allow the tonic to naturally replenish and rejuvenate your body. Please visit my website: www.TheEmpressSecret.com for more information about this new product. It will soon be available in the online store.

Determination, patience and discipline are what it takes for you to regain your health. There is no question of whether you are going to be healthy again; it is only matter of time.

For example, if you have been suffering from menopausal symptoms for years, it might take you a bit longer to get your body back to normal without HRT. If you are barely starting menopause and have minor symptoms, you may just drink 7-10 days of this formula and you will be fine.

It all depends on your condition and how consistently you are drinking the potion to give your body the continued, consistent nutrient. The key is consistency.

If you cannot do it on a continuing basis, then do not expect it to work. Ultimately, it is your body; you hold the ultimate power to take care of it.

Acknowledgements

First, I give the glory and honor to my Lord and Savior Jesus Christ. He is the one who led me on this journey with His purpose for me to do what I am doing. It is His grace and mercy that turned the darkest moments in my life to be the greatest blessing.

To Anika Janelle Pettiford, my beloved sister in Christ, my best friend, my mentor, and more than anything, my inspiration on my journey to seek out the Lord, to grow in Christ, to glorify our Lord, and to build the ultimate wealth for our Lord's Kingdom. I would have never even come close to where I am today without her, her endless love, support, and never-ending encouragement. Anika is like the hibiscus flower that radiates unbelievable shine and energy to everyone around her. My gratitude to her is beyond that words can describe.

To Mary Wilken, thank you for introducing me to Christ in Phoenix.

To my family, my beloved son Dylan. He is the most precious gift from God that changed my life and taught me how to embrace my experiences as a single mom to live my life to the fullest.

To Thomas Rider and his team, who made Empress' Secret Glow a dream come true with his graciousness, his vision and his believing in me doing something far more than just creating a drink.

To Nancy Hartwell, who edited my book with her detailed precision in grammar, punctuation, flow and structure and her superior professionalism to make this book come to fruition.

To Marcie Banda, who helped me get through some of the most difficult moments in my life with her strength, her wisdom and her endless love and support.

To Tom Robinson, who has always believed in me and offered his never- ending friendship and support.

To Kai Lin, who has always been such a role model in my life to look up to.

To all my beloved friends too numerous to list here, I am eternally grateful for all of you that brought positive impact to my life.

To all the women who have the chance to read this book: It is not a coincidence. It is a blessing and there is a purpose. The greatest gift I can share with you from my heart is for you to take control of your health and live life to its fullest with timeless beauty and irresistible glow while aging gracefully.

Blessings!

www.ingramcontent.com/pod-product-compliance
Lightning Source LLC
Chambersburg PA
CBHW070703290526
45790CB00001B/435